MAKE

WORLDS

David Krueger MD

HARD WORK MIRACLE PLAYBOOK

The Mind, Brain, and Performance Neuroscience of Sustained Success

europe books

www.europebooks.co.uk | info@europebooks.co.uk

ISBN 9791256971688
First edition: January 2026

HARD WORK MIRACLE PLAYBOOK

The Mind, Brain, and Performance Neuroscience of Sustained Success

To my favorite grandmother, who was always there.
Mamie's admonition became a mantra for my lifework:

If you're not having fun, you're not doing it right.

Contents

Introduction

If you can keep your head when all about you
Are losing theirs…
If you can trust yourself when all men doubt you…
If you can wait and not be tired by waiting…
If you can Meet with Triumph and Disaster
And treat those two impostors just the same…
Yours is the Earth and everything that's in it.

If, Rudyard Kipling

Barbara paused during one of our Mentor Coaching sessions focusing on her executive leadership strategies to mention that she would be distracted over the Thanksgiving holidays. She indicated with some embarrassment that each time she goes home to her family she notices the same problem. "We have a big gathering where my parents, brother, sister, and their families all come together for a holiday weekend, usually three days once a year. I resolve before I leave that this time will be different – that I won't get into arguments or struggles with my parents and brother and sister. I can usually last most of the first day, then something happens, and I lose it. I get in a fight with one of my family, which escalates to a fight with all of them. Is there anything you can do to help me with this?"

I responded, "I hear how frustrating it is when you want an enjoyable holiday with your family." She wholeheartedly agreed. I asked, "When you're in the middle of that upset and arguing with them, what is the age of that conversation for you?"

She needed no explanation to respond immediately, "Early adolescence. I'm 13 instantly and totally at that time. And I'm stuck there for the rest of the visit."

I asked her what she was aware of that specifically triggered her reactions. She described a particular look from her dad, a word from her mother, a gesture from her brother that would immediately provoke her to feel angry and criticized. Her reactive state of mind instantly transported her to that early adolescent time capsule.

I recommended that she schedule a time to do a brainstorming session with herself to reflect on the following:

- Column 1. List each specific *emotional trigger* with every family member.
- Column 2. Your *reaction* to each trigger thought, feeling, behavior, negative self-talk.

I suggested she schedule another brainstorming session with herself on another day to address two additional areas:

- Column 3. A 3-part *mantra* to get centered and present for each emotional trigger.
  - o A *cue* to initiate the process. (Barbara used the cue of touching her ring).
  - o A *focus phrase* to align the energy field of her brain (hers: "Relaxed and powerful").
  - o *Physiology* such as a deep breath for relaxation
- Column 4. An *ideal response* of thoughts, feelings, and behavior for each emotional trigger.

This proactive regulation of her state of mind included a new game plan for each situation.

She sent me the initial draft of her four columns. I emphasized that the purpose of the first two columns was to cue her radar to quickly recognize both the emotional triggers (Column 1) and the resultant state change to her age 13-time capsule (Column 2). Then to use her mantra (Column 3) to get grounded and centered to engage her ideal pre-planned response (Column 4) for each emotional trigger.

In our first session after the Thanksgiving holiday, she began the session by saying it was the best holiday she ever had with her family. There were times of challenge, even times when she would excuse herself for a private walk or go to the next room to get grounded and centered to create the response she wanted. She was immensely pleased with her work, as I was for her.

To further rewire this new attachment pattern, we reframed each of the previous emotional triggers as recognition of her family members' humaneness, and of her successful adulthood.

As Barbara noted, "That was incredible, but it was really hard work."

I responded, "I understand how hard and how successfully you worked. The only thing harder, as you already know, is not doing it."

In the last few years, we've seen revolutionary changes in our knowledge of neuroscience, psychology, and the performance sciences. We can apply this wealth of research to mindset regulation, stress mastery, and deliberate practice to achieve optimum performance under pressure. The operating programs of our minds and brains are not fixed but can evolve and transform. Just as scientific revolutions result more from asking better questions than from major discovery, better performance is also based on better questions. We can systematically rewrite mind software and rewire brain hardware to design new behavior and new performance stories. I will synthesize and integrate these new frontiers to help you become significantly more effective in your daily interactions, resilient to stress, and consistently attain peak performance.

The brain aligns its energy field to activate new connections through focused attention on possibilities and new experiences. Repetition then encodes new neural circuitry. We continue automatic and unconscious ways of operating until we become consciously aware of them. Because these processes are so embedded, we need a scientific way to understand them, and a practical system to encode new experiences to become new habits.

The principles and applied strategies in this book are informed by significant innovative research in neuroscience, behavioral economics, cognitive neuroscience, psychoanalysis, interviews with leading experts, and elite performers including SEAL teams, professional athletes, and corporate leaders. More recently, direct work as a Mentor Coach with performing professionals including actors and pro athletes, and extensive work with practicing professionals including physicians, attorneys, and financial professionals have all informed and honed the material that follows.

I have worked with everyone from concentration camp survivors to billionaires, professional athletes to business wizards, the unknown to the internationally famous. I taught medical students, psychiatry residents, psychoanalytic candidates, social work and psychology graduate students for 25 years. In the last 18 years, I have trained over 2,200 professional coaches on six continents and conducted online learning/continuing education courses for more than 21,000 professionals. I have directly trained an additional 475 licensed, specialty-certified coaches in my wellness, financial, and peak performance programs.

Hard Work Miracle PlayBook will challenge your existing belief system, strategically inform the development of what can be possible, and offer a science-based system for stress mastery and peak performance. Consider it a codebook for creating the algorithms of a performance story: a microsystem to regulate states of mind, and a macrosystem to construct an individual optimum performance story.

When you want to change a habit or create a new story, focus on the system, not only the goal. I will help you develop a simple, strategic, scientifically informed system to achieve and maintain exceptional performance.

Hard Work Miracle PlayBook will guide you through proven methods to both attain and maintain peak performance in your chosen field. Beliefs, facts, even attachment patterns are anatomical realities in the brain. Some of learning involves unlearning, a parallel process that is consistently addressed. So, you just can't input new information and expect it to overwrite a habit or pattern already existing. But change can occur as a scientifically informed and practical systematic process. A related aspect of this process involves navigating accompaniments of success such as wealth, power, and fame can brings can be equally challenging.

This informed and applied process becomes a hard work miracle.

When Dr. Helen Czerski was studying Physics at Cambridge, she was in her grandmother's kitchen looking at textbooks and charts of quantum mechanics. Her grandmother looked at her material and asked, "What can you do when you know that?"

Dr. Czerski has spent a professional lifetime answering that question and the unspoken follow-up question that she knew her Nana didn't say as she waited for the answer: "And why should I care?"

We're about to answer Nana's two questions, spoken and unspoken.

And I will help you systematically develop and implement strategies to achieve and sustain optimum performance.

For ease of discussion, I will use the term "Coach" throughout to refer to the guide for transformative change including mentor, coach, trainer, and leader. And the term "Player" as interchangeable with team member, protégé, mentee, and client.

SECTION I. PERFORMANCE PREPARATION

Two anthropologists were chosen to enter separate, essentially identical ape colonies where they would live and observe for a year, not communicating with each other. They and their respective Oxford research teams were chosen because of their remarkable similarities of personality, philosophy, and education.

When the two anthropologists emerged after a year to compare notes, they expected essential similarities but instead found remarkable discrepancies. One anthropologist, after an initial period of transition, was accepted by the apes, integrated into the colony, and achieved a unity and comfort with the apes. The other anthropologist never got beyond the social periphery of his colony, remained careful and vigilant, always seemed on the cusp of a conflict, and never reached a harmony.

The anthropologists could not understand the discrepant results or find any reasons. They and their teams puzzled for months until they finally found one difference. The anthropologist who was the uncomfortable, careful outsider carried a gun. His gun never showed; he never used it; the apes never knew he had it. But he knew he had it; he knew that if things got tough, he had an "out". The anthropologist who had no gun had a commitment: he knew from the beginning that he would either make it or not on his own.

In retrospect and reconstruction, each of their assumptions created the reality that they experienced.

Beliefs become predictors and confirm the reality that generates them. Beliefs take on a life of their own. Beliefs make up our identity. We work diligently to make our beliefs consistent with one another and with our identity. When we change our beliefs, we change ourselves as well as our identity. So, it is not a simple or easy matter.

We tell our story. Then our story tells us.

Neuroscientists estimate that from 90 to 95 percent of our operating system is unconscious. This means that the vast majority of our responses are based on established algorithms for behavioral, emotional, and performance patterns. This operating system ghostwrites beliefs, emotions, and behavior—the shadow stories on unconscious autopilot. As we repeat responses, the brain wires those as the default mode.

A script refers to the default mode of expectations, experiences, and responses that determine how we write our stories. Our expectations inform those brain patterns that result in typical—even stereotypical—responses to certain situations. The script for each scenario in our lives operates largely without conscious thought. At a family gathering or board meeting, we tend to sit in the same seat each time. We look over the menu each time and then order the same thing.

To understand the patterns and behaviors to enhance performance, we must examine the default mode, the script.

Systems are generally invisible to the brain. We do not detect the patterns that give order to the world, and especially to how our minds work. We are designed to adapt, react, fight, flee, and do various things for self-sufficiency and even self-actualization. Mapping the systems and the order that often lies hidden in our performance stories involve the invisible algorithms used to create what we think and do.

While our brains are coded to recognize the threat of a charging bull, we have no sensors to detect the carcinogenic effect of certain pollutants in food or in the air. So, one challenge becomes how to make the invisible tangible and concrete, to be able to understand and change the components.

Systems that occur over a long period of time are especially challenging, as the markers and the recognition of causal elements become elusive, such as with global warming. The factors that contribute to cardiovascular disease and a heart attack are patterns that occur over decades and perhaps only crystallize awareness with a myocardial event.

We do not innately have the neural radar for certain patterns. But we can systematically develop that radar, along with a plan for initiating and sustaining change, ultimately to make the plan a reality.

We'll explore how to create and encode new behavior side by side with unlearning old automatic behavior. The approaches to changing behavior that work also consider what this is doing to your personal story and identity.

The neuroscience of performance is based on a bedrock foundation of understanding both mind and brain. The anatomy of arousal involves a balance of neurochemicals that make up the essence of peak performance: dopamine, the pleasure neurotransmitter, norepinephrine, the neurochemical regulating attention and alertness, and acetylcholine, the neurochemical most involved in peak performance itself. We release acetylcholine at a critical time of new learning and brain neuroplasticity with focus and optimum learning machinery turned on. These three neurochemicals constitute the "DNA of peak performance."

Optimum arousal and full engagement can vary from person to person, even from situation to situation. Full engagement is specific to everyone in terms of state of mind, attainment, resilience, and regulation of that optimum state. Peak practice within that state develops the specific skills of performance. These distinctions emphasize the importance of self-awareness as well as knowledge of the mind, brain, and performance sciences. Coaches need to know everything players need to know and more: namely, they need to know how to catalyze change and transformation. And how to deal with extreme success themselves and with their players.

First, we'll discuss the basics of how the mind and brain influence performance. Then we'll lay out how, specifically, you can make use of this information.

Chapter 1. Performance Enhancement Basics: Several Minds, Two Brains, One Focus

1. Performance Enhancement Basics: Several Minds, Two Brains, One Focus

Several Minds

How can state of mind affect performance?

Put a rat in a maze and teach it where the food is, and the rat will find the food every time, because it remembers. But if you give the rat amphetamine (also known as “speed”) first, and then teach it where the food is, things change. Now, the rat can only remember while dosed with speed. Remove the drug, and the rat “forgets” where the food is. Provide the drug, and he suddenly “remembers.” It’s not really that the rat forgets or remembers; clearly, the memory is always there, or it couldn’t be accessed at all. What’s happening here?

Amphetamine triggers the body’s stress reaction. Because of this, the memory is formed in a state of stress, stored in that state—and the rat can only access the memory from that same state. Why? Because learning and memory are both state-dependent.

Have you ever forgotten someone’s name, tried to remember it on the spot, and failed? Only to remember it later, when the pressure was off. Same thing: the memory had to be accessed from a different state.

These examples illustrate the fact that there are different states of mind that are distinct from one another and have (in some respects) little or no overlap. It also explains why people can perform wonderfully while practicing or training—and then "choke up" or "stress out" under pressure.

Because brain chemistry affects the body, and vice versa, states of mind are mind-body states. It's as if each mindset is a piece of software, running on the body's system, with internally consistent emotions, memories, mental models and patterns of behavior. Switch it out with a different mindset, and everything changes: the way we perceive the world around us, how we process information—and how we perform.

Two Brains

Seth was a successful CPA who functioned brilliantly when focused on a single task—but that focus was easily derailed by external distractions, and he had trouble moving from one task to the next throughout the day.

To address this, he established daily and weekly schedules so he'd have a map for each day and could easily place any day in the context of that week. I suggested he keep his daily schedule on a Post-it note on the left side of his computer monitor, so he'd always know where he was. And a Post-it with his next best action or "NBA" on the right, so the next step was clear, and he could mentally prepare himself for it. I also suggested he update the NBA every hour, to ensure it was always current.

Making conscious decisions requires a tangible amount of energy (including glucose, which fuels the brain), so "automating" some things frees up the energy needed to make thoughtful decisions about other things.

Seth knew, at a glance, what his immediate (and next) task was. For his daily schedule, he took successful measures to counter distraction and increase focus:

- ☐ Determine the best times of day to do certain tasks (creative tasks in the morning, for example), and "protect" or reserve those times for those activities
- ☐ Eliminate interruptions/distractions by turning off his phone and cell phone ringer, email and message pings
- ☐ Schedule blocks of uninterrupted time to sustain the required state of mind
- ☐ Determine the optimum manageable block of time for any task.
- ☐ Write out the tasks for each day, scheduling them in one-hour blocks
- ☐ Prepare for each new task by focusing on the first specific step to be taken
- ☐ Cluster activities that require the same state of mind (errands, for example)
- ☐ Create a supportive work environment by, for example, removing or relocating distracting office items
- ☐ Advise colleagues and staff about non-interruptible time blocks, and schedule non-conflicting times for discussions, meetings, etc.
- ☐ Take a brief mindfulness/meditation break between tasks

Work-life balance requires boundaries, which—like the measures cited above—provide structure and increase effectiveness.

Two Brains: Top-Down and Bottom-Up Systems

At age 22, Chess Master Magnus Carlsen surpassed legendary Grandmaster Garry Kasparov and became the highest-ranked chess player in history. Though chess is a highly analytical game, and players are usually seen as hyper-rational and analytic, Carlsen is different. "I normally do what my intuition tells me to do," he says, "and most of the time spent thinking is just to double check."

The brain, essentially, has two independently operating systems with competing interests, or outputs: impulse and logic. The most pressing conflict we have is not between us and the rest of the world, but between these two systems in our brains.

We want to spend money now, but we also want to save for the future. We want to be healthy, but we want that cheesecake with strawberry topping. When we anticipate the purchase, the brain's reward center—the *nucleus acumbens*—releases the pleasure chemical dopamine. The brain's pain center—the *insula*—responds when we must pay.

System 1 and System 2 are descriptions of processes of functional operation of the brain, not localized anatomy or pathways within the brain. Both are brilliantly described by Dr. Daniel Kahneman in his book, *Thinking, Fast and Slow.*

System 1 (Bottom-Up)

The "Bottom-Up" system runs automatically, taking its cues from things like habits, impressions, previous experience, pattern recognition, and emotions. Its subcortical circuitry notifies the cortex (located at the top-front of the brain). This system was designed to keep our ancestors alive in a dangerous world where quick, impulsive actions were an evolutionary advantage. But today's world makes different demands, and we must implement focused strategies to enlist the "Bottom-Up" brain's cooperation in everything from self-awareness to deliberate planning.

This is crucial, because the Bottom-Up system operates automatically, and cannot be turned off at will. The intuitive, perceptive, often unconscious decision-making of this fast-thinking system relies on past experiences and pattern recognition. Left unguided, it may make errors of intuition and/or emotional origin—causing us to act without conscious thought. (Like snapping at a loved one because of something they had nothing to do with.) These kinds of errors can short-circuit executive decisions, athletic performance—and personal relationships.

Not surprisingly, the Bottom-Up brain is where most errors of bias and judgment arise. It's also the source of addictive habits that occur without conscious direction, things like overspending, over-borrowing, overeating, etc. Other issues are more subtle, like unconscious biases driving decisions that, if consciously considered, would go another way.

At times, good decisions are made by countering the intuitive, automatic system. An example is when you begin a skid on an icy road, steering into the skid instead of hitting the brakes.

System 2 (Top-Down)

The "Top-Down" System is the conscious, logical seat of self-control; in short, the rational mind. The left lateral prefrontal cortex is the part of the brain that deals with intellectual and abstract thinking, voluntary attention, consideration and choice.

Even so, our inherent patterns of belief, behavior, emotion and attachment originate in the Bottom-Up System and are executed by the Top-Down System. Unconscious decisions are made in the midbrain, then shifted to the forebrain, which makes those decisions seem conscious and logical.

Most of the time, the fluid synthesis between these two functional processes minimizes effort and maximizes performance. But some situations—learning, for example—occur when something new or different is introduced, requiring conscious effort. To maximize performance, we must recognize the situations in which we're likely to make mistakes, and the unconscious biases that can cause our brains to "ghostwrite" undesirable behaviors. We must also shift this recognition into conscious awareness.

One Focus

A tennis pro with an outstanding career found herself having trouble with her serve, just before Wimbledon. I asked her to take us frame by frame through her usual flow pattern when serving and then describe what felt different now. When she tossed the ball into the air, she said, she flashed to an image of her coach looking at her critically.

That brief instant interrupted a successful serving pattern that had become automatic. When she unintentionally moved from total reliance on her Bottom-Up brain—wired by tens of thousands of practice hours—to her Top-Down brain—where for a nanosecond she thought about what she was doing—she hit the ball slightly differently. And at her level, that tiny difference could be catastrophic. Once the problem was identified, she was able to return to her previous level of performance flow.

The brain is a pattern-seeking and problem-solving organ that processes our internal and external landscapes, so to speak. Pretty much every part of the brain is in constant communication with almost every other part of the brain. Optimum automatic communication happens when we're immersed in a performance mindset and a flow state suited to the task at hand. Likewise, this enhanced communication makes it easier to maintain that flow state.

The Power Is in the Focus

For our anniversary, my wife enrolled us both in the BMW Racing School in Greenville, South Carolina. The three-day course was a fascinating and masterful application of performance science, with professional racers guiding us through various driving challenges. One of the early lessons involved navigating curves and sharp turns at high speed. Because our brains follow our gaze—our focus—looking at where we want to go automatically guides mind and body to take us there. If, on the other hand, we focus on what we want to avoid, we usually wind up crashing into it. You get what you focus on, not what you want—unless the two are the same.

The unconscious mind does not distinguish between positive and negative, or future and past; it focuses solely on the here-and-now. Whatever you focus on—good or bad, near or far—is what your mind will move you toward. Attention serves to regulate emotion and determine which state of mind is chosen for any task. Successful performance means sustaining focus on one choice and ignoring others.

Noted coach and sports psychologist Harvey Dorfman tells a story from his teaching days: every time a new room was added to the school, it came with a new water fountain. The teacher across the hall from him posted a list of rules on the wall above her water fountain: "Don't stick gum on the spout," "Don't spit in the sink," etc. The rules were mostly ignored. The fountain in Harvey's room, though, had no posted rules—and was spotless. Harvey's lesson here was, don't demand what you can't enforce. Now, decades later, we realize there's another lesson here as well: focusing people on negativity tends to produce…negativity. And vice-versa. This most fundamental principle is from both neuroscience and quantum physics: you get what you focus on, not what you want. So, look at where you want to go, from the next curve or play to twenty years from now.

When a coach focuses on what not to do with a performer, it can become a prelude to a "choke." (More on this in in Chapter 9). Getting analytical, especially self-critical, interferes with the Bottom-Up brain's ability to sustain the performance zone, and instead to become an observer. The coach provides a safe, stable environment where the performer can practice, and even make new mistakes, without fear of criticism. The same dynamic applies to individuals, teams, and organizations.

For a soccer penalty kick, everyone is the same twelve yards away from a seventy-two-square foot target guarded by one goalie. When *playing to win*—when making the goal will result in a win—kickers are successful 92% of the time. Now consider the framework of *playing not to lose*: the team is down by one and you must make it to tie, and if you miss your team will lose. When that's the case, the success rate is 62%. Same distance, same target, two different mindsets that result in a 30 percent difference in success rate. In the threat mindset, expectations are high and there is the feeling of judgment—you can't make a single mistake. You play not to lose. The result is more anxiety and booting up of an entirely different mindset from the playing-to-win mindset.

Michael Phelps, the most highly decorated Olympic athlete in history, with 28 medals (23 of them gold), describes the significance of focus: "When I'm focused, there is not one single thing, person, anything that can stand in my way of doing something. If I want something bad enough, I'm going to get there."

Steph Curry, widely considered to be the greatest shooter in NBA history, has a specific spot he aims for when he shoots: the closest three net-hooks on the rim—which happen to be the same width as a basketball.

Our focus and our actions literally wire (and rewire) the synaptic connections in our brains. If we don't consciously focus our attention on what we want, the neuronal pathways in our brains will default to whatever it is we habitually pay attention to: bills, work, relationship problems, etc. This is why people sometimes get stuck in therapy; they focus on the things that are causing problems—but instead of then focusing on desired states or solutions, they re-engage with the problems. It's a vicious cycle that illustrates why a solution-based focus is more effective than a problem-based one.

Once a particular neural pathway has been formed, it can be strengthened by repeated use or weakened by disuse. The more it's used (and the stronger it becomes), the easier it is to find ourselves following or defaulting to that path again—and the harder it is to rewire.

An Olympic gymnast I worked with applied this principle in a powerful way. During her optimal performance state, when she was "in the flow," the briefest look at her opponent would break her concentration, her state, and her flow. To perform at her best, she had to sustain complete focus on her performance flow state.

Similar attention should be given to any performance, whether intellectual, athletic or artistic—immersing the performer in the entire sensory experience/awareness of the performance. This awareness comes when we are totally present and is essential to achieving "peak" or flow state. (Chapter 6 will cover deliberate practice while in-state.)

The most effective focused awareness is in and on the present moment. Any loss of that focus—even a single, momentary stray thought ("What if I mess this up?")—can "break" the state, resulting in diminished performance. Elite tennis players have learned to focus on the seam of the ball during their stroke, and to sustain that focus above all else. Other performers may focus on breathing, which directs attention to the immediate experience of being inside the body. Mindfulness meditation, which many peak performers make use of, focuses exclusively on breathing to target the wandering mind.

In *The Inner Game of Tennis*, author W. Timothy Gallwey stresses the importance of the inner game when off the court. When a player recognizes that learning to focus is more important than a backhand or forehand, they shift from the outer game to an inner game. "Instead of learning to focus to improve his tennis, he practices tennis to improve his focus," Gallwey says. When this shift occurs, it transforms concern about the results of the external game, into a focus on self-awareness.

Self-awareness and self-regulation are essential tools for remaining grounded and focused in the face of rapid, unsettling changes. One important aspect of self-awareness is the ability to recognize what you can and cannot determine—and to let go of the latter and focus your efforts on the former.

The principles of stress mastery and peak performance apply to all areas of sports, business, the arts, health, education and human relationships. As we grow more self-reflective and become better learners, we can more effectively write our own performance stories—in any or all these areas.

Selective Attention

How can specific focused attention enhance performance?

In the 2012 U.S. Open, Serena Williams and Victoria Azarenka were tied at one set each. In the third set, Serena found herself down by two games, at 3-5. Victoria was looking strong, but Serena was not prepared to lose. Slowly but surely—and rather amazingly—she fought her way back and won the last set 7-5. In a post-match interview, she said that rather than focusing on the high chance of losing the tournament, she focused her attention on a different question: What would it take to win?

Calculating that all she needed was twelve more points, she concentrated on that, point by point—focusing only on the current point in any given moment—until she won. Any thought of losing was a distraction, as was the next point. As was the point before. All that mattered was the present moment. There are systematic ways of creating, strengthening, and sustaining focused attention, which we'll cover in detail later.

Hyperfocus

Is it possible to be too focused?

In his book *Capture: A Theory of the Mind*, Dr. David Kessler describes how a stimulus like a person, place, object, smell or thought can seize our attention to the exclusion of all else, essentially hijacking our focus—and the mind itself. When attention narrows and gets stuck in a loop, there's a perceived lack of control, which leads to a change in emotional state.

Then, every time we respond, we strengthen the neural circuitry and make it easier to repeat the experience. As the neural conditioning grows stronger, it can feel like "something else" is in charge. The whole process can be positive—or cause pain and suffering. Either way, the process is something we're creating ourselves, moment by moment, while in the experience.

Hyperfocus can be avoided by establishing structure and boundaries (covered in Chapter 4). For now, know that it's important to have a firm end point or goal in mind for every training session or performance, to sustain orientation, to know the next step, as well as to know when to stop.

Chapter 2. Facilitating the Process of Change

Why do we resist change?
Even changing a story that doesn't work?
What keeps people from doing what they know they need to do for themselves?
Why will someone repeat behavior that doesn't work, often do it harder, and expect a different result? Even when it leads to lower energy, debt, plateaued careers, or disappointing relationships?

Part of the answer to why we resist change is in our minds.

We repeat the same story because it's our default mode: secure and predictable. It may be limiting or uncomfortable, but it's familiar. We repeat because we know how it will turn out, which creates the illusion of effectiveness.

A new story, on the other hand, generates uncertainty, trepidation. The easiest and fastest way to end this discomfort is to go back to the familiar: the old story.

People fail to change because they don't feel safe changing. Changing means leaving their home base of reality: the internal map that is synonymous with identity. We tend to return to our default mode.

A basic human need is certainty, especially certainty that we can avoid pain and achieve pleasure. The brain is a pattern-recognition machine that constantly tries to predict the near future. The act of creating a sense of certainty is reassuring. We repeat patterns, listen to the same music, go back to the places we've been, and order the same food because of the certainty of knowing exactly what will happen. Repetition, our collection of habits, masquerades as effectiveness. Change generates uncertainty. Even a small amount of uncertainty cues the brain's error detection mechanism, causing us to resist change. There is always the pull of the old and the fear of the new.

And part of the answer to why change is difficult is in our brains.

The hypnotherapist, Milton Erickson, told of a story from his childhood in which whenever it snowed, he would be the first to get up and go to school so that he could create a fresh path in the snow. He intentionally created a circuitous path, with zigzags and indirect turns. He noticed that each person who followed him followed the same path; at the end of the day, the path was well-worn despite its circuitous route. No one started a new, more direct route. No matter how many turns and twists, each person followed the path of least resistance.

This is how neural pathways are laid down in the brain: by early experiences and repetition until they are etched more deeply. Even if they don't work as well. Even if they're circuitous and require way more work. In most instances, change is perceived as danger to the nervous system, which will fight to protect you from doing the thing that you really want to do. This can show up as procrastination, perfectionism, isolation, defensiveness, unworthiness, or simple avoidance. Or simply as pushback from suggested change. The mind and brain both contribute to the pull of the old and the uncertainty of the new.

To think creatively, new neural pathways must be developed outside the cycle of existing experience. Stimulation for new insight is a circumstance where the brain can't predict what will happen next. The catalyst for insight is a novel stimulus: new information or new context.

This discomfort to move from the familiar old to the uncertain new becomes a challenge. The uncertainty of this newness can be read as evidence not to proceed, as intuition of a wrong choice. Or it can be reframed as a possibility, as a signpost of change and validation of progress.

Discomfort and uncertainty begin any significant journey. Our brains even have an error detection mechanism—located very close to the emotional center—that says, "This isn't normal," when we try something new. We'll discuss later how to use this mechanism as part of a powerful internal navigation system.

Two Fundamental Human Motivators

> *Nature has placed mankind under the governance of two sovereign masters, pain and pleasure.*
> Jeremy Bentham, Introduction to the Principles of Morals and Legislation (1789)

The desire to avoid pain and the desire to seek pleasure are we know twin forces of motivation that drive all human behavior. These two organizing principles of the brain for minimizing danger/pain and maximizing reward/pleasure become a fundamental way we inform and filter our perceptions. If we associate positive emotions or reward, we approach. If we associate negative emotions or pain, we avoid.

People will do more to avoid pain than to seek pleasure. Consumers are more concerned with not making a bad decision than making the best decision. We register twice as much pain from losing $100 as the pleasure we register from gaining $100 (loss aversion). Avoiding pain and its resultant inertia of remaining in the status quo generates the brain's tendency to create a shadow story. Think about how much of what we do is to prevent pain—paying bills, doing taxes, exercising, maintaining a house or a car, buying insurance. Since our brains are wired to prioritize survival over improvement, to prevent pain more than to seek pleasure, the wiring is designed more for protection than for success, fulfillment, and growth.

The need to avoid pain is biological. Our brains fight against change to avoid pain and uncertainty. Trying to create success by creating more pain unless achieving that success rarely works.

What we link inside our heads—the meanings that we give—determines our behavior. To change behavior, you must change what you link to pleasure and what you link to pain. The fact that the need to avoid pain is greater than the need for pleasure drives much of human behavior.

If you're not doing something that you want or need to do, you probably link more pain with doing it than with not doing it. If you don't have enough money or as much as you want, somewhere in your unconscious mind you may link greater pain to what you'll have to do to get it, such as work harder, or enter a high-pressure environment. The shadow story may not be conscious or logical, yet it becomes a powerful force.

If you experience any compromise of success in any area of your life, look at the approach (want pleasure) and avoidance (avert fear). Two questions for any procrastination or failure to engage a plan:

1. What is the greater pain if you don't do this?
2. What is the greater pleasure if you do this?

Pain avoidance results in a failure to follow through when you associate more pain with following through than with stopping. Seeking pleasure moves you toward every goal, personal and business. We'll discuss playing to win vs. playing not to lose in Chapter 10.

What neuroscience teaches us about facilitating change:

1. People have knowledge that affects how they hear and respond to new information.

   Existing knowledge is the beginning of new knowledge. It is where new learning starts, simply because it can happen no other way.

2. Existing knowledge is physical, real, and persistent as a neuronal pathway in the brain.

   Facts, beliefs, behavioral and attachment patterns are each an anatomical reality in the brain. Neuronal networks cannot be simply removed or easily overwritten by another fact. We can't present a simple explanation and remove an existing neuronal network from someone's brain. The pathways do, however, atrophy with disuse as other networks take their place. But it's an inside job.

3. If we ignore reality, it will get in the way of new information and change.

As we facilitate and co-create change, we must start where the person is, not where we are. We can't provide the tools for solving problems before they know what the problems are. This is why fixing doesn't work. You can't just list the reasons that an idea is wrong and expect that it will rearrange someone's neuronal network.

4. Partly because it is complex and personal and partly because it is subjective reality, people are not always aware of their existing knowledge.

Culture and Context in Performance Practice

The customs and practices of life in society sweep us along.

French philosopher Michel de Montaigne

Who do you practice, study, and brainstorm with?

We unconsciously download habits and behaviors from those around us and incorporate behavior patterns into our natural responses.

Our earliest habits are incorporated from the models and associated brain algorithms that we imitate from friends, family, schools, teachers, and peers. So many of these patterns are part of our unconscious operating system that we repeat without awareness, such as when to get married, how many children to have, the holidays we celebrate, even the money we spend on various items. We assume the body posture of the person we are conversing with. Invisible rules and unconscious scripts guide our daily behaviors. We imitate those behaviors without even recognizing it.

Several natural as well as designed studies show how likely we are to look to a group to guide our behavior, especially when we are unsure of how to behave. And we imitate the powerful—the idealized figures and heroes who represent prestige and status—to seemingly participate in those qualities. At times rather than feel helpless, we imitate and even take on the identity of those in power, assuming their perspective and purpose, such as in cases of Stockholm syndrome, as exemplified by Patty Hearst in the Symbionese Liberation Army.

The closer we are to someone, the more likely we are to imitate them. And the more time we spend with someone, the more likely we are to imitate some of their habits. Ryan Meldrum and associates found that the higher your best friend's IQ at age eleven, the higher your IQ will be at age fifteen. Factoring in natural levels of intelligence, these findings were true across all levels of intelligence.

Are there specific influences on individual habits that a social network can have?

We are all embedded in vast social networks of friends, families, coworkers, and more. Nicolas Christakis, MD, a professor of medicine at Harvard, studied social networks by following 12,067 people for thirty-two years. He found that clusters of friends show a "contamination" in the induction of obesity, unhappiness, drinking, smoking, exercise, and healthy diets. He shows how your location in the network affects your life in ways you don't even know, *even if you've never met them*:

- If your immediate circle of friends is obese, your risk of obesity is 45 percent higher.
- If your good friend becomes obese, it increases your chance of becoming obese by 57 percent in the same time.
- If your good friend's friends are obese, your risk is 25 percent higher.

This contagion effect of influences by others in a group can be powerfully channeled in a culture of a growth mindset, deliberate practice, and successful performance. It may be easier for those who are achieving similar things to support and praise those who are also achieving alongside them, in a team with a common purpose. Excellence in a team culture resonates with individual identity to become a powerful force when shaped by a wise and attuned coach.

These studies parallel the Framingham Study in medicine showing that clusters of friends show a "contamination" in the induction of obesity, unhappiness, drinking, and smoking. Possible explanations include that birds of a feather flock together (homophily) and that a norm or behavior can be spread from person to person by behavioral contagion and mirror neurons. "You change your ideal of what is an acceptable body type by looking at the people around you," Christakis says. We imitate the behavior of others, consciously and unconsciously, from what we invest to what we wear to our performance and success ethics. We find evidence for whatever mindset we choose and actualize those ideals.

One application is that when some in a group do a good thing, publicize it. If 80 percent of a team submits travel reports on time, be sure that the other 20 percent hear about it. If 76 percent of employees sign up for an automatic retirement plan contribution, publicize it.

Social networks can influence practices from wealth accumulation to wellness, and situations from market fluctuations to product adoption. Marketers recognize this contagion of popularity for commercial products by identifying thought leaders who spread the word and do viral marketing.

In a study conducted in San Diego, researchers hung four fliers on doorknobs:

One told homeowners they should conserve energy because it helped the environment.
One said saving energy was socially responsible.
One said it saved money.
The fourth said most neighbors in the community were doing it.

The researchers found that the households with the fourth flier showed the most change. Simply telling people that it's a good idea to recycle or conserve energy was the least effective.

Understanding the influence of social networks can help us understand phenomena such as:

- Successful team performance
- Health and emotions
- Market crashes and bank runs
- The spread of product adoption

- The spread of values and ideas

How can this contagion-of-success effect be applied to performance practice for teams?

Practice athletic endeavors, study with the best scholars, brainstorm with the most skilled people possible, and associate with a culture that represents your own ideals. A culture that excels at your desired behavior can enhance your own physical skill or intellectual development. As you individually pursue excellence, attunement to the habits of highly effective and successful people, especially in the areas where you want to excel, can guide to outcome. Engagement is sustained and enhanced by belonging to a tribe sharing interest and excellence. This influence solidifies when it aligns with your identity. *I am an athlete. I am a scholar. I am a leader. I am a reader.*

The culture determines a context of the behaviors that we view as attractive and desirable. We adopt behaviors that are regarded as praiseworthy by the culture we live in, those who fit with our tribe. We imitate habits of those close to us and whom we identify with as a member. Successful performance legacies can be developed and sustained in part through this epigenetic passing of culture.

The reason almost all smokers began smoking cigarettes is that their friends did it. Those who are most successful in managing to abstain from a habit are those who have a system and do it in a group, such as Alcoholics Anonymous or Overeaters Anonymous.

Each behavior is a joint effort of Top-Down and Bottom-Up Systems. A fundamental emotional decision by the Bottom-Up System is intuitive and automatic and then is processed by the conscious, logical Top-Down System to light on something that makes it make sense and seem logical.

Success is not an end point or finish line but a system for growing and transforming peak performance. A success system becomes a combination of self-reflection to create evolving improvement strategies and tools to build better habits.

Which sources have the greatest influence on players and player culture?

All sources in a culture are not weighted equally in terms of impact and influence. Influence is greatest by someone we see as most like us and what their predominant reaction is, as well as what specifically they react to.

Pick an influence leader and get buy-in, even collaboration, by first introducing an idea or new approach by asking their opinion. Then, collaboratively plan how to integrate this new practice along with endorsement and leadership in the team culture.

People are more likely to join in when people seen as most like themselves do so. At Latrobe University in Australia, studies were conducted to determine if corroborating evidence helps change minds by providing social reinforcement. The students responded based on how much like themselves they perceived the influencer to be. The influence leader can prime the pump for the team. This may not always be the star player; it may instead be the leader with the optimum emotional mindset of practice and performance—the player who sets the tone.

Do we perform better as we get closer to the finish line?

The objective is to get within reach of that finish line, because then it gives off a magnetic force. When you're close, you can feel that force pulling you, and you can use that force to get across. But just before you come within range, or just after, you feel another force, equally strong, pushing you away. It's inexplicable, mystical, these twin forces, these contradictory energies, but they both exist.
Andre Agassi

The vagus nerve is one of the pathways the brain and body use to talk to each other in unconscious conversation. Much of that conversation is about how we relate to others, as well as track social engagement, connection, and cooperation.

A welcoming situation or engaging conversation greenlights brain and body to prepare for a positive, friendly engagement. The vagus nerve is a pathway of the oxytocin system, the chemical of bonding and connection. It has been shown that the first few words of a conversation can boot up this response, or, alternatively, if the perception is of a threat or a need for defense, the yellow light activates a fight/flight mode mediated by the neurochemical system of cortisol and adrenaline.

Stephen Porges of Indiana University has studied and offered his Polyvagal Theory to explain the mind/brain/body mediation of these pathways. This work emphasizes that a synthesis of the brain and body working together, as well as co-regulation with coaches, can facilitate mutual emotional regulation, mastery, and superior performance.

The body and the brain collaborate in a complicated network of co-creative monitoring, regulating, and performing. World record-beating athletes do not slow down steadily over a long race as toxic metabolites increase and muscles tire; they instead spurt in the final stretch. Fatigue is both mental and physical, as researchers have shown again and again.

Goals become reference points, and we spend necessary energy to pursue and achieve them. *We become more motivated as we get closer to the finish line.* Donors become more generous in the home stretch when a target amount is within reach. It is simply more satisfying to compete, perform, or donate when we have an immediate sense that our effort makes a difference. Satisfaction enhances when we near and acquire a target.

The principle for a team: to create specific shared attainable goals. Then, the finish line must be reframed as a steppingstone to an even greater goal. Self-generated finish lines generate more motivation than those imposed externally. Goals can narrow focus and promote risk-taking, which can generate positive or negative effects depending on the framework.

The interplay between the finish line and the performer's brain is integral. For the performer to go the hardest, the performer needs to know when to finally stop—there needs to be a clear finish line. In the absence of that, the brain will conservatively regulate to hold the body back.

Fostering a Growth Mindset

British rugby coach Tony Smith lost his first fifteen games.

He framed each of the losses as trials, as a learning opportunity for both him and his team. During underperforming, he found a positive focus for each player as well as the group. He would identify one or two things for every person to work on after every practice and every game. This moved the mindset from problem and defeat to possibility and improvement. Additionally, each player recognized that Tony was watching everything they did while looking for ways to help them improve. A loss is only a loss when you don't learn from it.

He came to be regarded as one of the most influential and successful coaches in British rugby league history.

For elite performers, learning requires focus on their experience, including the learning style of the performer. Sports science incorporates a plurality of theories and approaches for communicating and teaching most effectively, recognizing the importance of collaborative communication and individual learning styles.

In preparation, leave nothing to chance. Attend to detail to focus on what can be determined and let go of what cannot. In preparation, leave nothing to chance.

Winners never lose focus on what they can determine, to accept the things they can't control.

Embrace the uncomfortable. Anything new and important begins with discomfort, uncertainty, and trepidation. Uncertainty must be embraced and tolerated.

The growth mindset of learning is based on a belief that basic qualities are cultivated and developed throughout life. You believe you can enhance and develop yourself. You become open to accurate information about talents and abilities. You use it to adjust and grow. Howard Gardner, in his book *Extraordinary Minds*, concluded that exceptional individuals with growth mindsets have a "special talent for identifying their own strengths and weaknesses."

If a coach says to someone, "You have great talent," it promotes a fixed mindset, as if talent is something you either do or don't possess and can be quantified to correlate with success.

A coach who says, "Congratulations, you worked very hard to achieve that," promotes a growth mindset to learn, improve, and achieve more. To believe that performance is related to innate talent or intrinsic ability will limit both effort and resilience. If talent or intellect are fixed commodities, then tenacious hard work will not sustain engagement.

How are beliefs incorporated into a growth mindset?

In 2018 an Italian gymnast began posting videos of himself in striking falls and crashes with the hashtag #GymnastsFallChallenge. Soon more than a thousand professional gymnasts posted their own experiences of mistakes to learn from them. The response was strikingly well-received, as ordinary people saw their everyday mistakes also made by these exceptional professionals. It also helped numerous people reframe failures as steps to their own personal success.

Beliefs are often unconscious, yet we can pay attention to the best indicators of beliefs: our behavior. We can nudge ourselves toward a growth mindset:

- Am I taking ownership of my mistakes?
- What can I learn from this?
- How can I improve?

In adulthood, whatever we experience we either create or accept.

How do you develop a performance growth mindset in players?

1. Think of a challenging, stressful experience or setback in which you demonstrated resilience and persevered to learn something important.
2. Create a story of that experience with the three components of story: challenge, development, and resolution.
3. Think about what the experience taught you and the model it provided for future reference for yourself and others.
   - What creative approaches and strengths did you employ?
   - What information, input, advice, or support helped you?
   - What did this challenge teach you about how to deal with adversity?

- How did this instance and scenario make you stronger?

A growth mindset views setbacks as inevitable and failures as catalysts for improvement and growth. The question is not whether you will ever have a setback, a challenge, or a failure, but what you will do because of it.

A growth mindset can create resilience through a coping style described by Edith Chen, psychologist at Northwestern University, involving a process she describes as shifting. Shifting combines four components:

1. Acknowledge stress
2. Learn about the source of stress
3. Recognize what can be changed
4. Determine what improvement can come from it

Persistence combined with positive framing can sustain optimism in the face of adversity: '"I think that things will get better in the future"; "I have a big purpose here and know that I will do better."

How can you recognize a fixed mindset?

Those with a fixed mindset try to make sure they succeed. A consuming goal is to prove oneself: in the classroom, in a career, or in a relationship. Each situation calls for a confirmation of intelligence, personality, or character. The repeated internal questions are these:

- Will I succeed or fail?
- Will I look smart or dumb?
- Will I be rejected or accepted?
- Will I be a loser or a winner?

- Will I attempt it without knowing I'll be great at it?

Yet with a fixed mindset, no amount of confirmation can dislodge the hypothesis of mediocrity or the need for proof.

A fixed mindset shares some of these beliefs:

- Intelligence is something basic and essentially unchangeable.
- You learn things but you cannot change how intelligent you are.
- You have fixed traits, so success is about proving that you are talented or smart.
- Problems indicate character flaws.
- Attempts to repair self-esteem include assigning blame or making excuses

How can optimism be enhanced and pessimism diminished?

Michael Jordan said, "I've missed more than nine thousand shots in my career. I've lost almost three hundred games. Twenty-six times, I've been trusted to take the game-winning shot and missed. I've failed over and over and over again in my life. And that is why I succeed."

Our mindset defines how we overcome failure and whether we learn from it to grow stronger. A growth mindset of positive approach may include:

- Truly believe that your efforts can improve.
- Informed practice will improve the results.
- Failure does not define but informs.
- A setback is an opportunity to learn.

- A setback is temporary and solvable.
- Look for information that shows the setback or any accompanying negative beliefs are factually incorrect.
- Look at how the setback can inform progress?

The way you regard the setback or failure rather than the event itself determines the next response. If the reaction is pessimistic, you may not try as hard the next time. An optimistic response will renew effort and enhance learning to improve.

Resilience Insurance

Several factors can tip the balance away from self-awareness and planning toward distraction or impulsivity. The imbalance can result in overspending, addictions, risk-taking, chokes, and other unforced errors. Understanding and planning can circumvent these issues and add to resilience.

Awareness of factors that predispose to distractions and compromised decisions can be remedied to provide resilience insurance:

- Depleted energy. When we become depleted for any reason, including the exercise of willpower, the tired brain yields more readily to temptation. When depleted, we tend to fall back on default mode and actions.
- Lowered blood glucose levels. Eight parole judges were studied for their decision-making regarding applications for parole. The average among all judges: 35 percent parole request approval. However, the exact time of each decision was studied in relation to the judge's

three food breaks: morning break, lunch break, and afternoon break. After each meal: 65 percent parole requests approval. Just before lunch and the end of the day (corresponding with lowest blood glucose levels): almost zero approval rate.

- Emotional overwhelm. The stronger the emotion, the more likely we are to act impulsively. Specific emotional triggers can instantly change a state of mind to generate emotionally driven reactions.
- High demands of self-control and concentration. Various activities that impose sustained self-control and concentration become depleting and have the impact of drawing energy away from an emotional bank account.
- Distraction. When we are distracted, we are more likely to lose focus on rational decision-making and react with a default pattern. Researchers Baba Shiv and Alexander Fedorikhin demonstrated that people succumb to temptation more frequently when the part of their brains that oversees deliberate thinking is preoccupied or overloaded.
- Abundance of choices. An excess of choices can overwhelm our bottom-up system to result in impulsivity or, at times, decision paralysis.
- Ineffectiveness or powerlessness. Subsequent attempts to counter helplessness or ineffectiveness often engage an action of anger, spending, eating or drinking to focus on a tangible action to effectively change a feeling. For example, one of the best days in the history of retail shops on Madison Avenue was the day of the stock market crash in 2008.

- Unconscious biases. Emotional states can activate preset meanings of unconscious biases. A study of sixteen years' worth of case files of judges with bachelor's degrees from Louisiana State University found that the judges gave significantly harsher sentences after LSU lost a football game it had been expected to win.

Shame/Blame vs. Growth/Transformation

Toni Morrison once asked parents about their children: "Do their eyes light up when they see you?"

This is a crucial question for any leader. Especially in the face of uncertainty, we are inclined to look for two things: the absolute and the closure. The finger pointing of blame conversation can accomplish both. In a culture of shame, someone or something in the organization needs to be blamed. This assignment of blame forecloses exploration of openness, learning, and growth. This reductionistic approach short-circuits exploration and new learning by assigning a cause and effect that becomes a black-and-white done deal.

Blame assignment discharges discomfort in the initiator and generates shame in the recipient. Discomfort, hurt, or helplessness discharged immediately by blame forecloses mutual exploration and the pursuit of more productive processes.

Organizations and teams with a win-lose mentality are most likely to use a shame/blame approach. Examine that hypothesis all the way to the end to evaluate whether it is working. Assess not only the wins and losses, but also the seasonal growth and lifetime contributions of each person in the organization.

A method of motivation involving shame can work for a little while, but ultimately the recipient will disengage for self-protection. Shame and blame can be replaced by mutual respect and transformative interactions.

The brain's mirror neuron system tracks emotions, unspoken intentions, body language, and especially states of mind, including confidence. The most instantly contagious experience from one person to another is state of mind, which has both spoken and unspoken emotional components. The brain of each member of a team will instantly register and resonate with the leader via mirror neurons.

A survey by the American Psychology Association found that 91 percent of children's stress is most determined by how stressed their parents are at any time. Their mirror neurons resonate with their parents' stress, spoken or unspoken, in an instant transfer. This contagion is faster than the fastest virus, going from mid-brain to mid-brain in a nanosecond. Same for organizations and leaders.

Engagement and Motivation Strategies for Optimum Learning

It takes one person to authentically create a safe environment of connection to change the trajectory of another person's life.

Shelley Barton Till

Researchers at the University of California, Berkeley, studied the value of positive feedback and its potential correlation with enthusiasm and winning. One person they followed in their study was NBA Hall of Famer Steve Nash, who was known for the energy and enthusiasm that were part of his leadership approach as well as his abilities as point guard. The number of times he touched a teammate as displays of enthusiasm or positive feedback per game averaged 239. This team-oriented enthusiasm and encouragement of teammates catalyzed a collective form of motivation.

Creating a collaborative alliance is always the first developmental phase of any working engagement whether individual or group. The alignment toward a collective goal enhances both the individual and the group. The initial step in building common ground with someone is an empathic resonance with their experience or challenge. State always comes first, then strategy and story. This empathic resonance co-creates a shared experience of the individual or group.

Collaborative engagement, tough conversations, and celebrations of success are all part of that shared experience. As with any focus on the system rather than just the goal, there are common elements of creating this shared experience:

1. Empathic resonance to engage to create a common ground.

   Empathize, clarify, affirm, and validate each person's feelings and intention without judgment or criticism.

2. Co-create a collaborative framework

   Creating the necessary trust for unfolding conversations and collaboration to be productive requires a safe and accepting environment. Some aspects of "saying whatever you need to say" may not be easy, but this developmental step of building a working alliance provides the framework of trust and safety.

3. Focus on the objective

   In situations that have emotional components and triggers, this sustained focus is especially important.

4. Regulation of state of mind

   The individual management of emotions and states of mind becomes important in determining performance decisions. The antithesis is impulsive action. Requirements include recognizing, owning, and assessing your own individual story, even as part of a group, to decide on the next best action.

5. Closure and gratitude

   Appreciate and express gratitude for the engagement. Agreement is not necessary, but closure is. Closure may involve a summary of the process as well as a resolution and, ideally, commitment to moving ahead.

   An important piece of closure is for each person to indicate the most important thing they are taking away from this process, as well as what they commit to doing going forward, within a specific time frame.

   In a group, this closing process may include each person's expressing in a single sentence the following reflections:

   - The most important takeaway from the experience
   - Each fellow member's most important contribution

- His or her action commitment based on the discussion

Focusing feedback on positive contributions has a powerful effect for everyone. The clear articulation of both the individual goal and the larger goal creates a motivating environment and a focus on the process of successful performance. The Gottman Ratio, named after the psychologist who conducted initial studies, states that a negative interaction has five times the impact of a positive interaction. This emphasis on the power of staying positive of supporting, believing, and caring about someone, has essential impact on successful performance. Alternatively, studies show that at a minimum, you have to offer five positive comments or interactions to a person for every negative one. Then the person being coached can build resilience and frame adversity as growth.

6. Follow-up

   Follow-up on the commitments expressed is the most neglected but most important aspect of accountability partnership with a player or group. It allows the process to continue with accountability to review both the process and outcome.

   As a result of this follow-up, there's much learning on both sides about what works, what doesn't, what may need to be revised, and how to create an ongoing process rather than a segmented event.

Negotiations are not about trying to convince but to understand. Trying to convince someone applies pressure, just as do arguments and threats. Optimum conversation is a collaboration to optimize performance.

This approach works significantly better than applying pressure or giving directives.

The Top Twenty-one Things a Coach Needs to Know

1. Listen with the intensity most people have only while talking.

2. Change is constant and inevitable; it is the resistance to change that generates most problems.

3. It takes two real people for a co-created reciprocity and collaboration to occur.

4. The roles of storyteller and listener unfold in the shared safe space of the coaching relationship, co-creating a new story.

5. Players know what they need, though not perhaps in conscious, logical, or daytime language, and will show us in the safe, co-regulated relationship process what it is like to be them, and what needs to be addressed.

6. We need to see the self that the player hopes to become, the evolving new story that sometimes gets obscured from view.

7. At times, a thought, feeling, or behavior is an answer to a question its creator has not dared to ask.

8. We must believe in the player until he or she teaches both of us why.

9. An authentic belief in someone activates their brain to create a state of mind that transcends usual thinking

and performance. People will do more than they thought possible when someone believes in them.

10. The architecture of trust silently forms while you talk about other things; the co-created new story gives oxygen to hope, highlights the relief and release of new experience, and pushes creativity to full flight.

11. A fact or a belief is an anatomical reality in someone's brain; a new belief or strategy can't simply overwrite what's already there. Change is a process.

12. We need to recognize the silent intent embedded in the compromised result to see the possibility camouflaged in the frustrating process.

13. Regulating states of mind is the most important success strategy. Each state has its own story.

14. Your state of mind will have emotional contagion for your players, colleagues, and staff.

15. Confidence is a state of mind influenced by repeated practice and co-regulated experiences.

16. Knowing what not to do is at least as important as knowing what to do. You may not always know what the next right thing is, but you can almost always know what it isn't.

17. Knowing how to reverse a behavior pattern is evidence that we truly understand it.

18. The most common thing that gets in the way of understanding something is trying to fix it.

19. Old stories must be mourned, and the self left behind. No matter how ready someone is to change, to

give up a long-practiced habit is like saying good-bye to an old friend.

20. You must have a new story to be in before you can completely let go of the old one.

21. To make change permanent, the new experience needs to be incorporated into one's identity.

Chapter 3. Co-Creating Successful Performance Stories

Half of this game is 90 percent mental.
Yogi Berra

The Influential Story Pattern

Consider these questions in coaching to engage players:

- *What initially causes someone to pay attention?*
- *What sustains engagement and attention?*
- *What do we unconsciously respond to when we hear or read a story that captures our attention?*

There is one answer to all these questions, coming from neuroscience, based on how our brains are wired to perceive and process stories. A story's secret is this: from the first sentence, *we must want to know what happens next.* When we want to know what happens next, the brain's pleasure system of dopamine fires and signals that intriguing information is unfolding. We pay attention and keep going.

A story is hardwired in our brains; it is how we strategically make sense of an overwhelming world and create game plans. When a story meets these hardwired expectations, it engages and becomes successful.

Nancy Duarte has studied the craft of storytelling and dramatic plot structure. By analyzing hundreds of the most famous, influential speeches of all time and testing different story structures, she discovered a story pattern at the foundation of the speeches. It is a combination of "what is" followed by "what could be" for several sequences. She superimposed the sequence of the patterns of Martin Luther King's "I Have a Dream" speech, Steve Jobs's well-known graduation speech, Lincoln's Gettysburg Address and hundreds of others. Each fit the same configuration pattern. Good parents, leaders, and successful coaches have known this for some time.

More than plot, purpose, winning, or losing—all abstract notions—the immediate impact of a story is its effect on the brain—the internal journey of "what happens next" to activate the dopamine system.

What three building blocks are common to all successful stories from effective marketing to bestselling novels to successful performance?

1. The Challenge
Find the challenge: the problem or desire.
From this knowledge, describe a situation as the person knows it: *what is.*

You are articulating what they already know and experience. This creates a bond of understanding—a common ground—between you and the person, and a readiness to hear your ideas for change.

2. The Development
The development of a story creates a bridge from the challenge to a resolution, a desired goal: *what could be.*

For this, it is helpful to know the person's external goal and what achieving that goal means—the motivation. An external goal is obvious; the internal goal involves how the external goal usually fits both purpose and identity.

3. The Resolution

Show how to co-create success. The mind and brain both seek closure. You help clearly and accurately associate a desired feeling or state with successful completion.

- Make it compelling and real—they will then authentically associate engagement with pleasure.
- We want emotionally but justify logically. Find the emotional reason—their reason—to engage now.

This three-part structure of challenge, development, and resolution that gives a story its shape can be applied to each component of deliberate practice.
Challenge. What is? Focus on the specific skill.
Development. What can be? Develop a systematic purposeful practice.
Resolution. Collaborative focus on how to achieve and sustain the successful outcome.

Neuroscience secrets of stories that are successful:

- We think in story, which allows us to envision the future.
- An active verb tense is perceived as more concrete and believable than a passive verb, because passive is more abstract. "I will …" vs. "I am trying …" Passive verbs include *is, am, are, were, was, be,* and *been.*

- When the brain focuses its full attention on something, it filters out all unnecessary information.
- Emotion determines the meaning of everything: feeling, state of mind, meaning attached, and behavior.
- Everything we do is goal-directed; objective self-reflection and self-evaluation can be challenging at times.
- We see the world not as it is but as we believe it to be.
- We don't think in abstract terms but in specific images. This means that anything abstract or conceptual must be made tangible, concrete and specific.
- If you can picture something, it's specific; if you can't, it's general.
- The brain is wired to resist change, even good change.

Some story checkpoints:

- *What is the point of your specific story?*
- *Can you sum up your story in a sentence?*
- *Do the plot, purpose, and theme of your story stick together to move toward the goal?*
- *Do the issues, themes, and plot answer the story question?*

When we read, tell, or live a story, the goal defines how we evaluate everything that we see and experience. If we don't know what we don't know, we will have no idea how to achieve it.

The Coach's Story

Consider these checkpoint questions as a coach:

- ☐ What do you most want?
- ☐ Do you know why you want it?
- ☐ What is your ultimate external goal?
- ☐ What is your internal purpose in achieving it?
- ☐ Is there a longstanding problem or fear to face to reach the goal?
- ☐ What is your biggest fear?
- ☐ What is your greatest desire?
- ☐ Where is your current performance story going?

The answers to these questions may help both coach and player reframe problems into possibilities, anxiety into excitement, and guide the direction of achievement.

The Question Launches the Story

Human systems grow in the direction of what they persistently ask questions about.
Dr. Diana Whitney

Dr. Diana Whitney, the founder of Appreciative Inquiry, was a guest in my Mastermind group and described systematic studies of Appreciative Inquiry in organizations that show three major aspects:

1. Focus on what works enhances what works: Ask about what you want more of, rather than about problems and barriers.

2. Focus becomes reality: A focus on possibility elicits a positive mindset; a focus on problems elicits a problem mindset.

3. Focus on what works awakens possibility: An "aha" experience that boots up a mindset that is more creative, synthetic, and integrative.

Appreciative Inquiry looks at how a person or organization can study and define the best that there is and then use that information to build on what is already working. People have more comfort and confidence to go further when they carry the best parts of the past forward.

Appreciative Inquiry can get much better results than seeking out or solving problems or giving the right answers. It is a complex science designed to not ignore problems but approach them from a different perspective. Appreciative Inquiry shows that collaborative strengths do more than perform—they transform.

The most comprehensive survey conducted on approaches to managing change and enhancing performance concluded that most organizations, teams, schools, companies, and families function on an unwritten misguided rule: to fix what is wrong and let the strengths take care of themselves. What really works is to align strengths so that weaknesses become irrelevant, and to know that some problems can't be solved, but have to be outlived by generating current successes.

Exploration of new possibilities recognizes the best in people or organizations to affirm strengths and potentials. The questions we ask plant seeds for the future. An organization's story, just as each individual's, is continually co-created and co-authored.

How does Appreciative Inquiry work at a brain level?

Evidence from brain sciences research demonstrates how a positive focus is immensely more powerful in aligning intentions and brain energy fields to bring about what we want. A confident, positive focus is contagious, and the leader's positive emotions are the most influential.

Eye tracking and brain imaging research found that peripheral vision literally and figuratively expands when someone experiences confident positive emotion.

Why not focus on problems initially in order to resolve and move beyond them?

Studies by Dr. David Cooperrider found that asking for problems boots up a problem-focused mindset in the recipient, while asking about success activates a mindset of success. The positive mindset fosters a dynamic force in the individual as well as in the organization's culture.

Four principles of the process of Appreciative Inquiry for an individual or organization:

1. Discovery. What is working best? Discovery of patterns of success creates a rich context for achieving more. Inquiry about what works well precedes visualizing the future. Start with discovery. We discover before we dream. Every positive question cues a mindset for exploration, a mindset to discover personal and organizational attributes, what people value, and how they hope to enhance the vitality of the group.

2. Dream. What is possible? Possibility aligned with purpose engages the entire person and team. An invitation to dream exercises imagination and looks at possibilities without limitations. The bolder the possibilities and vision, the bolder the attitude and the more successful the potential outcome.

3. Design. What options can we create? Study something at its best to further inhabit patterns of success. Attention to creating an ideal situation or organization crafts a clear purpose and set of organizing principles. Design a blueprint of relationships, roles, and responsibilities to further the purpose of an endeavor.

4. Destiny. What is your ultimate vision? Live the purpose, principles, and blueprint. Continue individual and organizational innovation to align with vision and values.

Appreciative Inquiry Tools

- Describe a time that was a high point experience, when you were most engaged and felt most alive and vibrant.
- What do you most value about yourself and your work?
- What are the core factors that give life to your organization at its best?
- Imagine yourself a year from now with everything as you wished it would be. Describe that.
- Imagine your organization a year from now with everything as you wished it would be. Describe that.
- What's the most important piece of new behavior to establish to move forward?
- For this big change, what is the first decision/behavior that would give you some traction in the process?
- What would demonstrate to yourself that you're moving forward?

How can a coach engage participation by the player and minimize opposition to instruction?

Asking a question will shift the listener's perspective to one of participant, of looking for answers rather than opposing a position or dictate of the coach. Once someone picks an answer, they are more likely to act consistently with that answer. A player is pulled by a question and by the answer much more effectively than he or she is pushed by an instruction. By responding to a question, the player gives more information to the coach and puts the process into an output channel. Asking rather than telling more likely inspires participation.

We commit to that which we help co-create.

Whether dealing with a terrorist or a suicide threat, the negotiator begins with asking how the person is, to make it about that person rather than about the negotiator. A demand or request makes it about the speaker, not the recipient. Asking a question to engage the thinking of the player creates a collaborative alignment with the player as point of reference. What the player thinks matters. When it matters, they will be more committed to their answer.

This is the first teamwork—the coach and player working together.

When I began coaching my son's team of six-year-olds, they were all playing basketball for the first time and didn't know anything about the game. I intuitively decided that rather than going over rules and a lot of instructions, we would have fun. If they were doing several different things, I focused on the one thing that was good practice rather than pointing out what they were doing that was wrong. Particularly when one player did something good, I highlighted this player's action and his experience of enjoying what worked.

Gradually, the number of best practices grew individually and for the team, and their pleasure grew because they learned how to be effective players.

Things that didn't work, like double dribbles, carrying the ball, and fouling were replaced by something better. As they regularly practiced the good stuff, the team became cohesive and successful.

Communication 101

4 Maxims of Communication

1. The person who makes a difference in your life is the one who listens as if he or she always knows who you are and gives it all back to you.

Each relationship combines two individual stories to coauthor a new relationship story. The unspoken assumptions by each person can facilitate or derail the relationship. Making explicit the hidden assumptions and implicit expectations becomes a crucial part of communication. To see the point of view of the other and to communicate that understanding, each must respect the other's point of view. Understanding and respect are not synonymous with agreement.

2. Ultimate freedom does not rely on another's response to determine how you feel.

Ineffectiveness of communication, simply feeling that what you said was not heard or registered by the other, may produce irritation or anger. Then the content of the discussion becomes more intense. The process that initiated the derailment—feeling invalidated —gets lost.

The simple step of repeating to the other what you heard prior to making your own point validates listening. You are then in a position to be heard more successfully. Your individual responsibility to co-author a mutually satisfying relationship includes the following:

- Mutual commitment to respect the other's needs and wants without neglecting your own
- Facilitation of communication
- Mutual negotiation on different points of view
- Explicit awareness of implicit assumptions
- Acknowledgement and understanding of needs and wants made obvious by relationship symptoms

3. The greatest vulnerability is daring to risk your best feelings.

4. The greatest satisfaction is risking your best feelings.

4 Steps of Communication

A basic human desire is to connect with another. The power within a relationship begins with a commitment to understand the other's experience, and to then collaborate to co-create an effective conversation.

1. Reflect back to the speaker what you heard him or her say.

This simple step assures the speaker of effectiveness—of being heard. If you're poised with a response rather than listening and reflecting, the speaker may feel a need to repeat; both speakers are then vulnerable to escalation of emotional tone. Knowing and respecting each other's point of view is the initial phase of a satisfying mutual collaboration.

2. Clarify by asking the next question.

Socrates taught us that really smart people ask questions rather than give answers. The detail may contain the feeling and the important aspects that otherwise would have to be assumed.

A large corporation's executive team huddled around a recording of the last presentation by the CEO of that company. They were playing it, rewinding it, playing it again. Each looked puzzled. The consultant asked them what they were trying to do. In his speech, the CEO had indicated that the organization should embrace more color. They each had a different idea about what color meant: Dress, race, decoration, language, stationery.

No one had considered simply picking up the phone and asking the next question, "What do you mean by color?"

3. Provide a context.

The context of any statement or meaning includes time, location, and framework.

4. Listen between the lines.

For someone who listens for facts, that filter will mean that the person stops listening when the speaker stops giving facts. When a very intelligent person listens for information, the communicator, to hold the listener's attention, must interweave information with the newness of what is being said. The speaker's empathic attunement to the listener includes creating a listening environment while providing information without losing the listener's attention.

Listen literally and closely to what someone says, and you will pick up constant clues about what is wanted and needed. Truth as well as reality is perception.

General Norman Schwarzkopf said, "I have seen leaders who stood in front of a platoon and all they saw was a platoon. But great leaders see it as 44 individuals, each of whom aspires, each of whom wants to live, each of whom wants to do good."

- Learn the stories of each of your players.
- Recognize the work and performance style of each player.
- Become aware of each player's optimum flow, the immersion that generates optimum performance from sustaining performance flow.
- Develop an awareness of each player's best learning, performance, and information processing styles.
- Celebrate small wins and personalize recognition.
- Ask questions and involve other coaches and players in making decisions.
- Share credit for improvement.

The bedrock of good communication is the foundation of a relationship with each player as well as the team.

Learning and Performance Styles

We all feel, process, and communicate differently, but there are fundamental styles that, when identified, can facilitate better communication. Optimum learning and performance occur when matched to the specific styles of each person. Although not all-or-nothing, each of these styles are consistent over time for each player.

• *Readers*

Some people learn best by reading and need to see a text or pictures to really comprehend material. They may do best when instructions and plans are printed and handed out. President John Kennedy was a reader who assembled an outstanding group of writers on his staff. Part of Kennedy's brilliance was in using these people and what they wrote to inform his decisions.

• *Listeners*

Some need to hear specific instruction even of well-written and diagrammed plans and strategies. President Johnson had attained his reputation and success as a listener. When Johnson kept the same people on his staff after he succeeded Kennedy, they kept on writing. Johnson derailed his presidency by not recognizing that he was a listener, not a reader.

• *Writers*

Some people learn best by writing. Encourage this output channel style of keeping a personal notebook to write reminders for certain players. Beethoven kept copious notes and amassed an enormous number of sketchbooks yet never looked at them when he composed. When asked about this practice, he said, "If I don't write it down immediately, I forget it right away. If

I put it into a sketchbook, I never forget it and I never have to look it up again."

•*Talkers*

Some people learn best by hearing themselves talk. This is a style I am quite familiar with. Verbally discuss strategies and responses with individuals and teams. I don't write because I have something to say, I write to see what I have to say. This and other books saw the first light of day when I talked to a specific imagined audience on a digital dictation device, and then had it transcribed.

• *Collaborators*

Some people work best in collaboration with others. Creative pairings and the dance of ideas are common for those who perform best in conjunction with others. Some collaborators work best as team members, succeeding in a system where ideas and implementation occur as part of a group to brainstorm strategies, ideas, and performance.

These predominant styles of learning constitute an important piece of self-knowledge and a way to facilitate communication.

Information Processing Systems

A kinesthetic wife asks her visually inclined husband how he feels about their discussion. His response, "I can see what you're saying," seems elusive to her. She asked about his feelings. She presses him to convert his model into hers, continuing to ask how he feels, what he senses. He repeats, "I can see exactly your points." They escalate. Rapport derails. She accuses him of being stubborn. Baffled, he retreats.

You can communicate better by appreciating the predominant mode of the other person. Developing empathy and establishing rapport with a player can be facilitated by awareness of the person's primary representational system.

At the beginning of a relationship, all three channels—kinesthetic, visual, and auditory—are active, both parties taking in a great deal of information, just as when traveling to a new country one is intensely taking in everything possible through all five senses. As a relationship progresses to developing and sustaining the connection, the intensity gives way to a default mode—the primary operating mode of auditory, kinesthetic, or visual. At this stage, communication issues become exaggerated.

Recognition of these distinct ways of processing information may be useful to consider in establishing and developing rapport and in fostering communication toward a common objective.

Auditory

Though not exclusive, an individual uses predominantly one representational mode. Those who take in information best through auditory presentation perceive experiences more in terms of sound and spoken word. They use phrases such as:

- I hear what you are saying
- It sounds good
- Within hearing distance
- I really want you to listen
- Tuned in
- Loud and clear

Visual

Those who primarily process in a visual way record and construct pictures or internal images of their experiences; they recall by snapping a picture into focus. Visual individuals will be inclined to say:

- Can you picture it?
- Bring this into focus
- Mental image
- I'd like to look at it
- I can see what you're saying
- It appears to me
- It seems fuzzy to me
- Short-sided

Kinesthetic

Kinesthetic individuals experience in a bodily way, and index information by sensation and feeling. Those more kinesthetic use sensory and bodily terms, such as:

- I need to grasp that.
- Come to grips with.
- Able to get a handle on it.
- Hand in hand.
- Hold on.
- Hold that thought.
- To be more in touch with...
- Start from scratch.
- I'll walk you through this.
- It slipped through my hands.

Neurolinguistic program researchers and practitioners have distilled some basic principles of recognizing the model and using it to facilitate communication.

- Recognize the predominant channel of processing information for yourself and the other person: auditory, visual, or kinesthetic.
- Respect the other person's model of the world, of perceiving and processing information along one of the three representational systems. One is not better than the other, just different.

• The observational skills of the type and meaning of communication is a necessary component of emotional intelligence.

• The meaning of the communication may be best indicated by the response that you get.

• The representational system, as well as the words, are only a symbol of the event, not the event itself. A map is not the territory. The model of your mind is not your mind.

• At times, the most important information about an individual is behavior.

• If what you are doing is not working, rather than doing it harder, think about doing it differently.

• Understanding this method of coding can facilitate more effective communication and collaboration.

Conversation Strategies

When Doc Rivers, then head coach of the Los Angeles Clippers, was asked what the most important thing was he does as a coach, his replied, "I communicate to my team. Not just collectively as a team, but individually. I must know where each person is in order to lead them where I need them to be." Doc later added that what he would most like to improve upon as a coach: "I would like to improve my communication."

What is meant by listening at different levels?

At a Retreat I conducted to train an organization to develop its own internal mentoring program, I did a demonstration Mentor Coaching with one of the Mentors. I asked her initially what she wanted to focus on in our session. She was vague, speaking in generalities about mentoring sessions with one of her Protégés with whom she had significant challenges. Unable to get her to focus more specifically on an agenda, I then asked what she wanted to walk away with from the coaching session. She still could not get beyond vague generalities.

After these unsuccessful efforts, I paused and asked if I could share a hunch with her to see if it would be helpful for us to consider. I wondered if she was experiencing the same reluctance as her client to open up and share a meaningful exchange, preferring instead to stay at a distance, even though feeling stuck.

She confirmed that this was true and said how embarrassed and reluctant she felt to share any of her struggles in front of her peers. She had never participated in a demonstration coaching or had witnesses for a mentoring session. I told her that I understood entirely, and that it wasn't easy to share intimate details about an experience in front of someone else, and especially a number of peers.

I suggested that she consider her experience as an exact read of her Protégé, that the reluctance that she was experiencing with me and showing me precisely replicated what her protégé was trying to tell her, through the process of the exchange, rather than consciously and with words.

She immediately understood what I was saying and recognized that that was precisely what was happening. She then began to open herself to discuss aspects of the engagement that were challenging and now more accessible to her and collaborated with me on strategies and ways to address this issue with herself as a prerequisite to addressing it with her Protégé. Previously immersed in her own discomfort, she was unaware of her unfolding interactive attachment pattern that replicated the one between herself and her Protégé.

We came to see that when she felt confident about herself as a Mentor, she could be totally present with me. She then knew that she could help her Protégé evolve his story and dare to risk some of his experiences with her. Her parallel of both the process and the attachment pattern in the engagement with me allowed both of us to see how her Protégé was teaching her exactly what it was like to be him. And how she was then demonstrating in vivo with me what he needed.

What are the essentials to effectively engineer change?

When Terry Fox ran the Marathon of Hope, the cross-Canada run of 3,339 miles, he ran with a shuffle and a hop because he had an artificial leg. Yet he managed to average twenty-four miles a day and complete the race in 143 days. Immediately on completion, he was asked in an interviewed, "How did you manage with your challenge when you were tired and still had thousands of miles to go?" His simple response: "I just kept going to the next telephone pole."

1. Specify the next step.
   Avoid the abstract and the global. Some is not a number. Soon is not a time. Act healthier is not a strategy.

2. Focus specifically on the next immediate issue.

3. Make changes tangible and concrete.
   Construct a yardstick or a map to determine where you are and where you are going so that you can

measure progress along the way and tell what is detour and distraction.

4. Make progress measurable.
   Demystify the journey: Have a specific destination, to tangibly focus on the next step.

5. Make progress visible.
   Establish small, specific, attainable milestones that are visible, with celebration of each small victory.

An example of shrinking a task to a tangible next item is how Alcoholics Anonymous challenges its members to "one day at a time." It shrinks the change to a manageable, foreseeable specific action. A small target leads to small victories, the cumulative experience of effectiveness and mastery.

What strategies are there for the oppositional player?

When a change does not occur, such as with a player and a new initiative or execution, the tendency is to push, encourage, give more information, and pressure change behavior. To perhaps give more examples and explanation and apply more pressure to change. The natural assumption is that more reasons and arguments, or at least more force, will be all that is necessary. Most often this is exactly what doesn't work, and entrenchment and pushback pressure is heightened. Resistance builds by telling someone what to do.

An alternative strategy is to identify what is preventing change from happening and to collaboratively remove that barrier. In this way the coach is a catalyst of change with less energy, no resistance, and toward a collaborative goal. The best way to persuade someone is to encourage them to persuade themselves. This is the coach as a catalyst.

Parents know that it does not work to tell a child what they must do, such as what they must eat. Being given certain options, pre-chosen by parents, allows the child to choose whether to eat the broccoli or chicken first, whether to have the milk out of the yellow or blue cup. This bypasses pushback and opposition to co-create a choice along selected pathways to optimize results. Provide selective choices. Guide the player with selective options so they can experience agency—their own effectiveness—in choosing how they get to where you want them to go.

Guided options shift the focus to choice rather than agreement or capitulation and allow the player to retain a sense of control. People will commit to what they help create. The player becomes a stakeholder in both the action and the outcome. Catalysts start by asking questions. This approach establishes an open, growth mindset of possibility, gathers more information, and increases buy-in to the process of successful resolution. Having a player actively choose in the process helps them to feel they have more active input in the process. The menu is a limited set of options from which the player can choose, all of which focus on performance enhancement.

If the coach presents one directive and asks the player to buy in, the player likely pushes back to focus on flaws or drawbacks in that method. By presenting two or three options, players can focus on the sense of agency to make their choice become the successful one. Having too many choices—more than two or three—can result in decision paralysis and reversion to the default mode of the old way of doing things.

By providing a choice, questions shift the listener's role to collaboratively making decisions on potential answers rather than countering a mandate. This shift moves from reasons to oppose to a search for answers. When it becomes their own answer, it becomes their own success.

The first step is always to put yourself in the listener's shoes rather than moving directly to a strategy or resolution. This is the beginning of trust and collaboration. State before strategy and story. Helping the listeners come to their own conclusions offers the best possibility of engagement and successful outcome. Rather than beginning with persuasion, begin with understanding.

Focusing on only one step shrinks the change to make that step specifically attainable. When there is a sticking point and things seem hopelessly stuck, find a point where there is agreement and proceed from there. Finding common ground on which to build trust and understanding allows moving ahead together.

When there is disagreement, ask for less. When the team is stuck or resistant, begin with an influencer, or a more flexible member already most closely aligned with your position as coach.

What are the fundamental essentials of communication that the coach needs to be aware of to be effective?

The biggest block to personal communication is man's inability to listen intelligently, understandingly, and skillfully to another person.
Carl Rogers

Perhaps the most fundamental skill any coach can possess is knowing how to communicate with players. Not just to guide deliberate practice and performance enhancement, but to allow players to open about worries, insecurities, and fears. Because every player, artist, or business professional will have a slump, a setback, or a choke. The coach needs to know how to hold a mirror to the player for both to look together, collaboratively, as they figure out what to do next and better.

1. The coach's state of mind.
   With self-regulation and self-awareness, the coach needs to be grounded and centered, accessing a confident state of mind.
2. The communication itself, verbal and nonverbal.
   Both participants, when engaged and connected, can communicate at an authentic level, optimizing mutual self-regulation.
3. The player's system of perceiving the communication.
   The coach needs awareness of co-regulation to establish a grounded connection with the player, leading the way by modeling an optimum state of mind for the player to receive all information and to process it with full internal access.

In all three of these steps, the coach sets the tone and establishes the model for the immediate communication.

Verbal and nonverbal language, along with self-awareness of a regulated state of mind, all become important.

A study of college level tutors was titled "Why Do Only Some Events Cause Learning During Human Tutoring?" The best learning occurred at the point that the student reached an impasse and was ready to receive input. The biggest gains were from engaging a particular challenge or struggle at the time it occurred. And not functioning for the student. Tutors impaired learning when they provided answers and support too quickly, and particularly when the student was not at an impasse.

A challenge can prompt deep learning. We learned as parents to not take over and keep tying our child's shoes. It would have been easier to keep doing that, but the child learned frustration tolerance leads to learning. Perhaps even more importantly, the child looked into the mirror of the parent to see that the parent believes the child's innate ability to learn and to persist. This model becomes internalized as a belief in oneself, and formed a pattern of persistence, the groundwork of resilience.

Asking a question rather than giving information opens engagement to join collaboratively to co-create answers.

Important reminders about communication:

- The coach and player both send and receive communication.
- Both use verbal and nonverbal language in their communication.

• A lack of understanding of the meaning of the message for both sender and receiver can create disruption.
• Mixed or unclear messages can create confusion.
• Understanding and respecting the communication process can be significantly beneficial.
• Repeat what the other just said to convey understanding. "What I hear you saying is…" Then the receiver can respond to correct or agree—either way, feeling heard. This establishes a common ground on which the receiver and the communicator can proceed.
• Coaching is teaching.

And there are times when usual collaboration doesn't work. One year when I was head coach of a boys' basketball team, one of the guys I'll call Pete had difficulty regulating his emotions and controlling his behavior in basketball games. We had discussed this, individually and as a team, but the behavior persisted. After three technical fouls in the first two games, when a technical was called on Pete in the third game, I called a timeout and motioned him over to talk privately. "Pete, that's the next-to-last technical foul you will ever get as a member of my team," I said. He looked at me with an astonished expression and knew I was serious. I then said, "I believe in you and want you to still be my starting center if you decide."

For the remainder of the season, he never got that next technical foul and came to be a leader and second highest scorer on the team.

How can the coach foster psychological safety and a foundation of trust with the player?

He taught life.
Bill Walton on the coaching style of John Wooden

John Wooden offered a fundamental view about a coach's major responsibility: "He should remember he's there to teach. He should remember he's there to get a player to learn." This emphasis on the coach's responsibility to teach goes beyond recruiting great players and guiding winning performances. The wise coach recognizes that the players are not simply outstanding performers but are fundamentally human with balanced emotional, family, social, and economic dimensions.

1. Start by asking questions. This does two things: it gathers information and creates a participant in the process to make it collaborative. Ask, don't tell. Guided options shift the focus to choice rather than agreement or capitulation. A select menu redirects focus to help someone retain a sense of control. If a mentor coach presents only one idea, the subsequent focus by the player probably will be to look at exceptions or reasons that it may not be the best way to proceed. Presenting two but no more than three options, all of which will enhance some aspect of performance, will increase buy-in by the player. Asking the right question has more power than giving people the right answers. Appreciative inquiry can get much better results than seeking out and solving problems.

2. Focus on possibilities. We know from appreciative inquiry that establishing an optimum performance mindset of possibility begins with the power of positive framing and asking generative questions. Ask about possibilities rather than problems. The nature of the conversation with the player will have profound impact on expectations, the relationship, and subsequent accomplishments. The player moves toward the images and belief that the mentor coach has in mind. When you look for problems, you will find problems. When you look for solutions and leadership, you will find possibilities. A positive framework and asking generative questions create a positive engagement and performance.

3. Be mindful of the first words you speak as a mentor coach. We know from the neuroscience of conversational intelligence that the first words spoken trigger a neurochemical reaction in the listener to boot up a specific mindset that then processes the remainder of the conversation to determine meaning and significance. A conversation that begins with what is perceived to be authoritative, critical, or adversarial remarks activates the brain circuitry of fight and flight. The player experiences anxiety or distrust and closes down for self-protection. A conversation, however, that begins in a collaborative mode activates the brain's neurochemical system of oxytocin, the system of bonding and connection. This initial perception of a collaborative, trusting response induces listening without judgment and paying full attention to the speaker and frames the remainder of the conversation as a joint endeavor. The player then feels safe and understood to develop trust.

People will commit to what they help create. Be clear about what behaviors and practices you want more of to focus on that. When the coach connects with the player as a person, this care about t needs and concerns becomes a foundation of a trusting relationship on which everything else is built, including performance. Communication by the mentor coach is not about giving information, instructions, or directives but about a collaborative co-creative engagement for individual and team development and performance.

The most fundamental skill any coach can possess is knowing how to communicate with players. Not just to instruct deliberate practice and facilitate performance enhancement, but to allow the player to be able to open up about worries, insecurities, and fears at the right time.

Confidence Is a State of Mind

Olympic gold medalist Noureddine Morceli of Algeria said, "When I race, my mind is full of doubts—who will finish second, who will finish third?"

Confidence is a state of mind built on the foundation of experience, knowledge, and the cumulative experiences of mastery. Confidence does not mean unafraid, invincible, or unquestioning. It means that whatever challenges or obstacles occur, many of which cannot be predicted, you can create a belief system of knowing that you will create a successful outcome. Preparation and knowledge framed in that belief become self-fulfilling.

A lack of confidence, negative self-talk, doubt, or feeling like an impostor are all indications of an immediate need to get grounded in a focused, optimum mindset.

Accessing a Confidence Mindset

There are three potential ways to actively access the state of confidence:

1. Physiology
    - Stand up
    - Breathe strong
    - Say "yes!!"
    - Move deliberately with confidence. "I can do anything."

2. Control your mental focus.
    - What you focus on determines how you feel. If you focus on how things might not work out, you will lack confidence.
    - We then experience whatever we sustain focus on.

3. Change core beliefs.
    - Success begins with beliefs. Beliefs become real, then reinforced.
    - When I can imagine it, I can achieve it.
    - When I am committed, there's always a way to make it work.
    - To change outcome, change belief.

Use of your physical body can effectively put you in a state of confidence no matter what you were feeling previously. Confidence is not something that you have or don't have but a state of mind entered by the way you speak, move, or gesture.

Success most often has to do with two things:

- The state of mind of confidence that you engage an endeavor
- How you maintain an optimum performance state under pressure-inducing circumstances

Creating and sustaining an optimum performance involves these steps:

1. State: Your mindset will determine both your story (including confidence) and your strategy.
2. Strategy: A systematic way to practice and perform.
3. Story: Your belief system that guides what you see and do.

How can you prime your mind and brain to prepare for an anticipated situation and establish a mindset of confidence?

Here's how not to do it:

By yelling at his point guard for missing that wide-open teammate in the corner, a coach has probably ensured that it will happen again (Alexander Wolff, Sports Illustrated).

In the game Taboo, you have a target word on a card you have drawn that you want your partner to say given your single-word clues that aren't accompanied by gestures. Also on that card with the target word are a half dozen words you cannot use. The words that would make it too easy. Think about how hard it is, once you have seen those six words, not to say one of those words. If you say one of those six taboo words, you lose the point. Often what you should not say can frame and dominate thinking to make it hard to get beyond the taboo words to offer reasonable clues.

A common perception is that the best way to get employees or players to perform is by pointing out mistakes, making threats, or being intense. While negative emotions grab attention, a positive focus works considerably better to develop confidence as a mindset and the associated aspects of loyalty, bonding, personal development, and commitment to a group.

Reframing mistakes as information to learn may help not only learning but also coping skillfully and resiliently the next time. And it can help you relax into the self-acceptance that contributes to confidence. Mistakes, equanimity, keeping calm, carrying on, and experiencing effectiveness often initially precede confidence. And then to recognize that you have become more of who you truly are. Courage is not the absence of fear but the will to proceed despite it.

In high-pressure situations, the ability to remain focused and sustain a state of mind of confidence determines outcome to a significant degree. In research examining 185 venture capital pitches (like those seen on Shark Tank), confidence as manifested by calmness and eye contact combined with passion was the greatest predictor of outcome—greater than combined content, expertise, and experience. Sustaining a balanced and confident state of mind ensured the most favorable outcomes.

Priming of mind and brain to prepare for an anticipated situation establishes the foundation of a mindset of confidence. Here are seven strategies for successful priming for confidence:

- Have a mantra for grounding and centering.
- Ask yourself positive, powerful questions to induce serotonin.
- Recall a time of similar accomplishment.
- Identify moments of significant confidence, a feeling of "I can do it" or "Whatever it takes."
- Focus on connections with important others to activate oxytocin response.
- Create mental imagery of success to live into.
- Cultivate a circle of support people and coaches.

Is there a way to sustain and enhance confidence as a mindset?

Confidence is a state of mind that can be shaped by informed action. Here is a game plan to enhance both confidence and performance:

- Repeat attempts with adjustments for learning.
- Review and possibly recalibrate results.
- Adjust and move forward.
- Fail fast.
- Assess consistently.
- Adjust.
- Move forward.
- Leave your comfort zone.
- When in doubt, act.

An interesting aspect is that those who are overconfident do not alienate others or necessarily appear narcissistic if they genuinely believe their own confidence even though it may be overrated. On the other hand, fake confidence doesn't work well and appears as narcissistic, alienating others. Purity of action, wholeheartedness, and positive energy are also the attributes associated with confidence in Buddhist teachings.

Three components on the blacklist of confidence include dwelling in mistakes, inability to shut out the outside world (wanting to please people), and letting setbacks linger. Confidence can be compromised by overthinking, people-pleasing, and dwelling on defeat.

Consider the approaches that have been linked to diminished confidence:

- Being thin-skinned and preferring to be liked rather than respected
- Being afraid to say no and abandoning your own needs
- Being unwilling to make someone mad by asking for more money
- Ruminating about a criticism or negative comment rather than seeing it as a self-statement of the speaker or writer
- Taking the blame for things gone bad and crediting fate for successes
- Overpersonalizing a setback and undermining confidence

Section II. PERFORMANCE PRACTICE

When I was in the singles ski lift line at Steamboat Springs about to advance to the chairlift, an instructor behind me who had five kids all about age five asked me if I would mind if two of them rode the chairlift with me. Of course, I welcomed the opportunity.

As we got on the lift, the little girl next to me had a somewhat awkward seating and seemed to slump a little bit as we were riding and talking. As we got close to the end of the lift, she said in a very timid voice, “I’m scared to get off.”

“I understand,” I said. “Do you know who Laurie Hernandez is?” Laurie had won a gold in the team event and a silver on the balance beam in the Summer Olympics. The little girl looked at me and said, “Yes.” I asked her if she would like to know what Laurie did when she was scared about performing her gymnastics routine. She immediately said, “Yeah!” I told her that Laurie did three things. She pictured herself doing a perfect routine, a vision of exactly how she would perform. Then, the instant before she began, she took a deep breath to breathe in relaxation and breathe out any tension, and said to herself, “I got this.”

My new little buddy seemed interested in this and sat just a bit more upright. As we were a few seconds from getting off the lift, I asked her what she would say to herself as she got off.

“I got this,” she said in a timid, hesitant voice.

I nudged her. “Say it like you really mean it.”

Then, in a voice that seemed to channel all her five years into someone I wouldn’t want to meet in a dark alley, she said very confidently, “I got this.”

As she skied out of the chair perfectly, she stopped and turned to look at me from about ten feet away. At the same instant, we both did a one-inch air fist bump. We both smiled, and then she skied off with her instructor.

Breakthroughs in neuroscience, cognitive psychology, and behavioral sciences have created radically new ways to guide performance and map success. Mind- and brain-based strategies integrated with performance science can have dramatic effects on the way we interact, lead, and perform. Performance enhancement principles and systems form the template of deliberate practice for peak performance.

The brain has a unique way of writing into code and creating complex algorithms that may be consciously inaccessible but can generate intricately developed stories of behavior and performance. Understanding and rewriting these patterns leads to significant enhancement.

Information has never been sufficient to generate change. If information were enough, we would all eat mostly vegetables, work out every day, be thin, and have a lot of money saved up. And several librarians would be billionaires. But information is not the foundation of change. The process must be addressed in a stepwise systematic manner to result in transformation of each person’s operating system, performance, and core identity to make the change permanent.

This section will apply evidence-based learning and deliberate practice strategies for developing peak performance systems. Science is about understanding patterns, the fundamental laws and principles that form the foundation of our lives and world. The brain is a pattern-seeking organ, yet many of the methods of facilitating change are contrary to the way the mind and brain work. It's not about having all the answers, since most of our operating system is unconscious and not directly accessible but about having an informed framework for asking the right questions and an evidence-based system for optimum performance. This section presents systematic ways to reprogram mind software and rewire brain hardwire for peak performance.

We'll apply two proven systems to address optimum performance:

1. The Neural Conditioning Program is a performance microsystem for managing emotional triggers and rewiring planned, ideal responses for peak performance. The Neural Conditioning Program addresses an evidence-based model to generate optimum responses at a behavioral and brain level. The simple four steps will help you effectively manage states of mind and strategically plan optimum performance. This systematic architecture of state of mind regulation guides you to rewire your brain for new behaviors for optimum performance.

2. The ROADMAP System® is a performance macrosystem for deconstructing and understanding personal performance to systematically write new code for mind, brain, and behavior. ROADMAP is an acronym

for the seven steps of a scientific and systematic way to deconstruct and understand personally created stories and to strategically create new behavior. Understanding behavior and performance algorithms couples with a methodology to generate a new, enhanced performance story. The development of corresponding new identity becomes the bedrock that allows this transformation to become permanent. The ROADMAP System offers a blueprint of performance story construction to understand and address the mind and brain creation of thoughts, feelings, and behaviors organized into an accomplished performance story. A ROADMAP System for Performing Under Pressure illustrates an application.

Chapter 4. Learning and Practice Strategies to Develop Peak Performance

Logic and sermons never convince.
Walt Whitman

Transformative Learning

A distinguishing feature of great coaches is that they develop strong, healthy relationships with their athletes. It is clear that these coaches genuinely care about the well-being of their players beyond their performance.
David Grand and Alan Goldberg

Legendary basketball coach John Wooden, who won more national titles as head coach for the UCLA Bruins than any other college basketball coach in history, did not talk to his players about winning and losing. He didn't talk about beating opponents. Instead, he focused on what he felt that he and his team could determine: effort and attitude in the present moment. And letting go of what could not be determined, including the abstract result of winning.

With this internal point of reference, each player learned to focus on the immediate aspect of what they could determine moment by moment. This left no room for focusing on comparing themselves with others, avoiding losing, or doing anything other than complete immersion in this moment of practice and play. Wooden emphasized the things that each player had total determination of effort, attitude, growth, improvement, focus, and state of mind. Ten national championships in 12 seasons testify how this philosophy works.

What are the steps of transformative learning?

Here are the basic aspects that we'll apply to a series of performance-related practices:

1. Begin with a positive mindset.

How you think and believe about your learning dramatically impacts effectiveness and application. Changing how you think changes how much you can learn. Whatever you attempt to learn, a positive approach of optimistic engagement anchors the remaining process. The belief that you will not be able to do it results in not being able to do it. The most effective learners take charge of their own learning and do not let obstacles be sufficient reason not to proceed. A growth mindset looks at any specific challenge to determine optimum possibility, process, and outcome.

2. Establish a system for practice and learning to include:

- Set specific goals, limited to two to three at a time.
- Create goals that are challenging.
- Set achievable stepwise goals, as each achievement further motivates the process.
- Determine a target date for each goal.
- Identify specific needs in the learning process and set about addressing them.
- Identify holes in what you need to learn rather than working on what you are already good at.
- Challenge yourself with tasks just outside your ability.
- Interweave different tasks in the same learning segment.

3. Actively engage in processing information vs. passive acquisition.

Ask questions and find other ways of engaging a task to process and respond with the new learning as part of its acquisition process. Testing yourself is one of the best ways to learn new material or new skills. Testing yourself offers better learning probability than rereading or redoing, because testing yourself requires retrieval and use of the output channel for new material or skill. Test, practice, consolidate, learn.

4. Identify optimum information sources that will challenge you, especially a coach.

Seek out different points of view and alternate perspectives. Engagement with additional informed points of view can stretch and challenge your default assumptions and behaviors.

5. Address physical activity, nutrition, and sleep as important learning and performance components.

Brain and body both need to be optimally functioning. Learning always includes optimum sleep because the hippocampus transfers information that is deemed worthy of retaining to long-term memory during sleep.

Is there a proven best way to learn from mistakes?

Michael Jordan spoke of a lesson he learned from his University of North Carolina coach Dean Smith. Jordan would return in the offseason to talk and play pickup games in Chapel Hill. He described to Smith his frustration with his Chicago Bulls teammates' attitude toward losing. He regarded their attitude as uncaring compared with his practice of staying in the shower for up to an hour after a loss to replay everything he did wrong. At other times, he would sit in the locker room with a towel over his head, reviewing the images of mistakes. He assumed his teammates didn't care as much when they would shower and leave.

Smith wisely reflected to Jordan that for him to become an elite player, he should give himself ten to twenty minutes to reflect on a bad performance to learn everything he could about it during that time. Then he should think about the superb basketball he would play in the next game or think of positive things in his life other than basketball. He emphasized to Jordan that continuing to relive his mistakes would lead to reproducing them.

We now know from neuroscience how absolutely accurate this is, that we get what we focus on, and the more we review, remember, and visualize, the more it etches those pathways into the brain.

Exceptional people deal with mistakes and failure in two steps: the immediate step to learn from it and self-correct and the second step to wipe it from memory. To reflect on a failure or mistake to learn from it is distinct from using it as an anchor or a point of reference. The worst thing any performer of any sort can do is to dwell on mistakes and create negative judgments from them.

Self-talk is also important in this respect. Don't dwell on the negative but create an optimistic hope and plan for the future. The growth mindset is to look for what can be learned and done differently and to develop a commitment to do it.

How can we use our knowledge of the mind and brain to create psychological tools for optimum performance?

San Antonio Spurs all-star Tim Duncan said, "When you have to stop and think, that's when you mess up." Honing your mind needs the same attention as honing your craft or skill. Performance mindset is the framework of performance skill and execution. To perform optimally, an engagement of flow is necessary. To focus on a specific aspect of that performance during the performance of that skill interrupts the flow. For example, when a soccer player focuses on what side of the foot a kick occurs on, performance is compromised as the athlete moves from the practiced state of flow. Anything that interrupts that flow, whether a distracting thought, a spectator, or thinking about how to do some aspect, can compromise performance.

Practicing under the conditions of performance creates a brain-grooved experience of automatic performance. Whether preparing for a game, a performance, an exam, or a presentation, the way you practice will determine the way you perform.

What is the role of emotion in learning?

Learning happens best with emotional integration, whether positive or negative. When an experience is emotionally relevant, new information is engaged and retained to a much higher degree. There are two simple tests that the hypothalamus subjects to any information to decide its relevance and worthiness of remembering: emotional engagement and novelty. These two experiences activate either the reward or threat response.

We understand, learn, and remember best with stories that help us make sense of things. We learn in the context of connection with others and the stories that are co-created. Authentic and transformative relationships develop optimally with the learner in a collaborative context. This context is the antithesis of only providing information or instruction.

Transformative learning is distinct from conveying accepted information, purposes, beliefs, values, and judgments from the coach. The goal is to create independent thinking and learning, to construct personal meaning, and to develop effective self-functioning and self-authorship performance stories.

The process of self-reflection, autonomous thinking, and personal performance development facilitates brain structure changes during a learning process. An initial step for the learner is to become "critically reflective of their own assumptions underlying intentions, values, beliefs, and feelings" (Dr. Jack Mezirow).

Which works better, rewards for positive performance or punishment for bad performance?

Much evidence supports the finding that rewards for positive performance work significantly better than punishment for bad performance. Remember from neuroscience that we get what we focus on. Response—positive or negative—heightens the probability of repetition. Many insightful parents have figured this out from their children: whatever they respond to is sustained or enhanced.

Because of our mind and brain wiring and function, this strongest form of negative learning comes from negative experiences and the engrams they create. Yet, aversive learning is essentially an ineffective way to train positive behavior and should be saved for those few situations designed to inhibit undesired behavior.

What framework will most enhance motivation to learn?

Motivation is essentially internally driven to fulfill core human needs of competence, autonomy, and relatedness. Definable goals enhance motivation to achieve them. Specific strategies of measurable steps to the goal enhance focus and attention in the process.

Perfectionistic standards undermine performance for two reasons. "Perfect," like "more," is to not have a goal—there is no end point for either. To continually strive for something that is just out of reach ultimately diminishes resilience and the desire to pursue. Second, the perfectionist is probably looking for the approval of others, creating a vulnerable reliability on a response not determined by the performer.

Emphasis on avoiding mistakes often creates mistakes. Since you bring about what you focus on, attention is drawn to the wrong thing. The perfectionist takes a hit when mistakes happen, diminishing both motivation and future performance.

What do the best performers do that set them apart?

We know that motivation is enhanced the closer we get to the goal. An important aspect of sustaining motivation and developing resilience is setting things up so that we see consistent and concrete signs of laddered improvement. Small, specific steps validate effectiveness, the most basic of our human motivations, and sustain motivational energy.

The antithesis of *perfectionist* striving is *excellence* striving. The pursuit of excellence incorporates mistakes as a learning process, and point toward challenging, flexible, and realistic goals. The antithesis of control is mastery. Mistakes are not failures but opportunities to learn. Success becomes improvement rather than perfection. Problems become learning tools rather than setbacks or inconvenience. Acknowledgment of problems initiates problem-solving. Feelings are not avoided but initiate self-compassion. Regardless of gender, age, race, or culture, self-compassion enhances self-awareness and performance.

Is there an art and science to goal setting?

Goals can enhance motivation by focusing on what to specifically accomplish and prioritize.

Goals that show the least positive impact on performance are ones that are either exceptionally easy or exceptionally hard and barely attainable. To set goals very high and rationalize that even if you don't reach them your achievements will be significant can backfire. This strategy fails to consider the fundamental motivation of effectiveness, the need to experience mastery day to day. We basically don't sustain motivation for goals that we know we won't hit.

Ideals form the compass, and goals become the map to determine specifically where to go. The plan—the strategy—integrates the two. Performers who align with their ideals—their core identity—train harder and work more consistently. They make better choices in the face of adversity and are more likely to persevere.

Context is important. Surround yourself with like-minded people. States of mind and energy fields (which have a common denominator) are contagious.

What can sustain immersion in a performance zone?

In sports competition, elite athletes often feel that they operate without effort, perhaps can anticipate what an opponent will do, and at times feel that time is slowing down coupled with a sharpened vision. In this zone, executive control portions of the brain become more active. Especially for fast-moving sports such as tennis, basketball, or baseball, visual focus becomes even more important for quick snapshots. Focus on a simple and specific activity essentially bypasses emotional and mental patterns to remain at the sweet spot of the performance mindset.

For other activities, such as endurance sports like long-distance running, cycling, business, or surgical procedures, performance is enhanced by relaxation response techniques before performance. For example, a runner or biker focuses on steady and repeated leg action to sustain the performance zone.

The sweet spot in the performance zone is a state of mind of performance where you don't think about it at all but enter the state for automatic immersion in the developed skill. A consistent preparation system to enter the zone, whether for an athletic, intellectual, or artistic endeavor, can vary significantly from individual to individual.

What is the most common performance leadership fallacy?

Dr. Daniel Kahneman relates a story of teaching instructors in the Israeli Air Force about the psychology of performance. He emphasized that a positive focus on skill development for performance works better than punishments for mistakes. A seasoned flight instructor challenged Dr. Kahneman's research, indicating that on many occasions he praised flight instructors for good performances and that the next time they performed that maneuver, they usually did worse. He also indicated that after he would scream into a cadet's earphone after poor performance, the cadet would then do better. From these experiences he concluded that punishment works better than reward.

Kahneman acknowledged that the situations where the instructor praised an outstanding performance were likely to be followed by a performance that was less than outstanding. And that punishments were more likely to be followed by improvements. But Kahneman explained that the reason wasn't necessarily that punishment is more effective than reward. More likely, it was due to the second-most common leadership fallacy (after the notion that if you provide enough excellent information, you will effectively cause someone to change their minds or buy your product): that the best predictor of the next response is the *average* of past responses: the *regression to the mean*. An outstanding performance by all odds will be followed by what is most average for that person. Odds are that a poor performance will most likely be elevated in the next response to that person's average, reading as an improvement of the performance. The inference that the instructor's words were causal would be incorrect.

In sports and business, a coach or executive will praise excellent performance and most likely see a subsequent decrease in performance the next day or play. And the coach or executive who chastises for poor performance will then seen an improved response. The understandable conclusion for both is that the intervention was the cause. We consistently seek causal explanations and infer one even when it isn't there to end brain dissonance and create mind closure.

Any extreme group or individual performance will regress to the mean over time. Kahneman uses the example of an intervention with depressed children. An intervention with very depressed children over a three-month period, whether it's regularly giving them an energy drink or having them hug a cat for twenty minutes a day, would result in improvement. But it's not because of the drink or the cat. It's because this is an extreme group and they will eventually approximate the mean, which is to become less depressed. The same depressed children will get better over time even if they did not consume an energy drink or hug a cat. A study using a controlled group with any intervention is necessary to truly discern causality or, at the very least, relationship. Correlation and causation are common confusions even in academic research.

Is there a best way to end a performance (besides winning)?

In an interview with Andrew Garfield, who played Spider-Man in two films, about his current role in the Broadway play Angels in America, nominated for a record eleven Tony Awards, Willie Geist asked "How do you even get out of that character?" A compelling question for such an emotionally and physically demanding role in a two-part Broadway play. Garfield replied, "There has to be a ritual to get back into yourself. Humphrey Bogart used to go sailing. For me, it's people who I use as anchors back into who I am. I also do a little ritual every night where I write a letter and sign out as the character and back into myself." He describes how he does this every night for the days when he performs.

When I began playing basketball with my son and daughter in the driveway many years ago, we would never end on a miss. They had to make the last basket they shot before we stopped. Later, when I coached their basketball teams, each player had to make the last basket he or she shot before we ended practice.

Somehow, I knew intuitively that endings made a difference. Even brief, seemingly meaningless endings of our driveway basketball or our Tuesday night team practices before the big game on Saturday. Later I would learn of Kahneman's research on peak experience that found that the two times of the most impactful experience and subsequent memory are the moment of greatest emotional impact and the ending.

The experience at the end of a sequence or practice is most vividly remembered (Peak End Rule).

Retrospective assessments are weighted by experiences at peak moments and at end moments. These two times create more vivid and lasting memories.

The ending of any behavior, of any practice, is perhaps the most important aspect of the entire sequence. The ending is vital because we tend to remember the ending more than any of the other phases. To develop a skill, a habit, deliberate practice needs to incorporate a satisfying ending. The ending may simply be reinforcement, a self-imposed reward to enhance the experience. But more than anything, it is the experience of effectiveness and the resultant mastery that reinforce behavior.

My son, two years older than my daughter, also taught me about the importance of a performance state of mind. With his being the first team I ever coached, when he was age eight, we would gather as a group at our home gym the day of the game, shoot briefly, and go over the few rudimentary plays that we had. The team would then all pile into my car (remember, this was the era before mandatory seat belts) and drive to the gym while listening to "Eye of the Tiger." A raucous repetition of the song, in which they all sang along at high volume, got everyone into the spirit before the game.

When I later coached my daughter's all-girl basketball team when she reached age eight, we began each practice the same way, with a little inspirational talk, teamwork, moving directly into basics, and then scrimmage. It didn't work. They were distracted and didn't seem to respond, as if they were there for something besides basketball. I was baffled. As I listened to them and observed more closely, I began to sense what I had missed. Basketball was the content of the practice, but their state of mind focused on the process of being together, playing together. While I was urging them to concentrate on being competitive, they just wanted to enjoy themselves and each other. Soon enough, we began each practice sitting in a circle on the court, just talking. That was their warmup, and it worked; they played better as a team. Same thing for pregame warm-up: we all piled into my car and gossiped on the way to the game.

How strange yet wonderful, I thought, it must be to be a girl. And to apologize when you foul an opponent was never a consideration for me. My daughter still contributes to my continuing education by giving me four granddaughters.

What social interaction factors most positively affect optimal learning?

Social cognitive and neural sciences have demonstrated some fundamental components of various social interactions that most positively affect learning and achievement:

1. Effectiveness

How does a player feel after interacting with you: validated, valued, appreciated, important? Or do they feel invalidated, unimportant, unappreciated? This experience addresses the basic desire of effectiveness in interaction. Significance, the need to feel important, special, and unique, can be incorporated into an ideal of achievement and peak performance.

2. Certainty

Our brains consistently attempt to predict the future, to anticipate what will happen next. We consistently scan, intuit, and engage predictable hypotheses of predictability. When a coach is transparent about what happens next, or about expectations, this engages the certainty of knowing exactly what to do to be more effective. This creates a sense of mastery, the experience of that most fundamental of human needs, effectiveness.

3. Autonomy

Effectiveness from an internal point of reference defines the experience of mastery. Rather than being an extension of someone else's point of view or directive, having an internal point of reference generates a sense of autonomy.

4. Connection

We experience connection in various ways: friendship, intimacy, prayer, or simply the desire to bond to another. This fundamental need of connection applies to important others in the group or the team.

5. Fairness

The experience of being treated fairly is a personal emotional response, enhanced by transparency. When we perceive fairness, the brain releases a pleasure chemical. When we perceive unfairness, we feel pain as unfairness triggers the reptile, primitive part of our brain that mediates threats and survival. The perception of unfairness often results from some variation of being pushed out of a valued community, being left out or treated negatively in an important relationship or situation.

These social interactions directly address the fundamental human needs of certainty, effectiveness, significance, connection, growth, and contribution. Peak performance occurs when these fundamental needs are met in fulfilling, optimum ways.

As human beings, we all have the same needs. Our differences become the vehicles we use to fulfill those needs. People will violate their ideals, their values, to meet their needs. When fundamental needs and ideals align with strategies and goals, optimum learning evolves for peak performance.

Endurance as Mindset

Talent is insignificant. I know a lot of talented ruins. Beyond talent lie all the usual words: discipline, love, luck, but most of all endurance.
James Baldwin

How can you change the limits your brain places on your physical performance to break through to a new level?

Endurance becomes a mindset expectation of deliberate practice for exceptional performance. Training brain performance algorithms for performance execution determines the default microdecisions automatically executed in the flow state of performance. A crucial component of training is examining the narrative about both potential and performance. The belief of limits or the belief of optimum successful performance can become lived experiences.

In the last decade, paradigm-altering research has contributed significantly to performance science and execution. The physical barriers of performance endurance are considerably more elastic than once considered. Physical barriers are determined more by the brain than by the body, and an important component of both training and performance includes integrating brain and body aspects. Every aspect of training becomes brain training as well. When brain training is integrated in deliberate practice, it becomes part of the flow of performance.

Researchers at Oxford Brookes University, in Great Britain, found that pain tolerance increased by 41 percent in a group who reframed pain as the validation of improvement in performance. They found that greater physical fitness was not the crucial factor in increasing pain tolerance but how that fitness is practiced and endured.

Neuroimaging studies across several types of sports conclude that enhanced internal awareness allows elite athletes to prepare for unpleasantness and pain. A study in *British Journal of Sports Medicine* confirmed that reframing expectable pain as signpost of progress improves practice resilience.

Creating Enjoyment in Performance

You guys have had an unbelievable year; the winningest team in Kansas basketball history. Think about that. You are the winningest team in Kansas basketball history. Nobody can ever take that from you. Nobody. So if they can't take that from you, basically we got nothing to lose tonight. Nothing. But we got so much to gain. The reason I feel so confident about us winning is because we don't have to change one bit who we are. For thirty-nine games, you displayed how hard you're going to play, you displayed how you're going to guard, you displayed how you're going to rebound, and you displayed how we're going to steal extra possessions.

All we have to do is be ourselves. Let's go have some fun.

Bill Self, head coach of the University of Kansas, spoke these words to his team before the NCAA Championship Game in 2008 against the University of Memphis, which resulted in an upset victory over favored Memphis.

Enjoyment of practice develops a skill with the love and pleasure of the learning task rather than to focus on the defeat of an opponent. Just as we use memories to forget, the point of the focused effort in deliberate practice is to lose yourself in the flow of the experience.

The hard work of change is closely tied to pleasure, connected to the brain's reward system. The release of the pleasure chemical dopamine with the enjoyment of success also modulates gene expression critical to brain development and integration of that activity as part of an identity. The joy and pleasure of effectiveness become the emotional fuel to sustain and reward achievement.

How do you bring out the best in a performer when your team is going through a challenging time?

- Remember that you establish the mindset and mood of the team. You establish the model that they download and operate on for individual and collective performance. Each member of the team will download your belief, optimism, and mindset and actualize them in their culture and performance.
- Foster confidence as a state of mind and group standard.

• Participation by each player to the collective effort and success of the team.
• Respect and celebrate each individual performance contribution.
• Talk about the player's perception, evaluation of performance, and subjective experience. Invite talking about whatever is on their mind that may relate to their performance. Establish a relationship of openness and transparency.
• Use information to guide within a framework of skilled coaching and performance rather than as simply a means to persuade.
• Clarify the distinction of your decisions and your belief in the individual decisions within the domain of each of the performers.
• Schedule regular one-on-ones.
• Schedule team meetings to talk about the process of collaboration, teamwork, and culture. Keep the team informed of relevant aspects; each member is important enough to be kept abreast of what is happening and what you are thinking.
• "Never change a winning game. Always change a losing one" (Bill Tilden, number one tennis player in the world for seven years).

What is the role of willpower in practice and performance?

I have a good friend who decided to pay top dollar for a hunting dog. He got his new buddy as a puppy and grew to love this dog. He had him professionally trained by one of the best in the business.

When we were together, I asked him how things were going with his new hunting companion. He looked immediately dejected, slumped a little, as he told me how disappointed he was. He said, “I take Lex out to my ranch, and we’re both excited about our outing. As soon as I let him go, he runs a straight line at full speed until he’s exhausted and conks out. I have to go get him and carry him back every time.”

Lex reminds us of the importance of the dosing, timing, and titrating of practice and performance of several skills. This kind of fatigue is not the best purposeful practice. With exhaustion, we lose concentration, make errors, and generate bad habits.

How do you keep going in purposeful practice despite setbacks?

Dr. Benjamin Bloom studied the childhoods of a number of experts in diverse fields. A consistent finding was that their parents used strategies to keep them from quitting. One of the most consistent examples for several of those studied was a time when they were injured or sick in some way that kept them from practicing in their future field of expertise for some period. When they then resumed practicing, they found that they were much less accomplished than they were before and understandably discouraged and wanted to quit. Uniformly, the parents indicated that they could quit but suggested that they first needed to practice enough to get back to where they were. Once they have done this, and gotten back to where they were, they realized the experience of effectiveness and the belief that they could continue to get better. They saw their setback as temporary.

What are some common influencers of willpower?

Willpower can be influenced by several variables, from practice to awareness of things that deplete it, such as stress, sustained mental effort, or low glucose. Exerting willpower requires brain energy and needs to be developed with practice and regulated with sufficient restoration. (Stanford Psychologist Kelly McGonigal, The Willpower Instinct). Hunger, fatigue, and psychological conflict deplete willpower stamina. Children who develop the highest level of self-control as children have less than half as many health problems as adults compared with those with lower levels of self-control. Willpower is one of the most important predictors of success in life. (Duke University)

Efforts of self-control and practice willpower become tiring. The more you must force yourself to do something, subsequently the less self-control you have for the next challenge. Various activities that impose high demands of self-control and concentration become depleting and have an impact by withdrawing energy from emotional bank account. This phenomenon of ego depletion has been studied by psychologist Roy Baumeister, who found that all variance of voluntary effort – emotional, physical, or cognitive – draw from a shared pool of mental energy.

When someone becomes depleted from a task, they succumb more quickly to the urge to revert to an old model or to respond impulsively. The result of this depletion may have various expressions:

- Overspending on impulse purchases
- Abandoning a healthy diet
- Lowered threshold for annoyance or impulsivity

- Performing less well on cognitive tasks and logical decision-making
- Persisting for less time in challenging tasks

Mental energy is more than a metaphor. The nervous system consumes considerably more glucose than other aspects of the body, and mental activity is expensive in glucose currency.

There is another approach that takes no energy and results in 100% success. This approach does not take motivation into account, does not consider the benefits and the liabilities of doing or not doing something, and takes no energy to engage this process each day.

That solution is simply to structure a plan and stick to it. The plan needs to have a daily commitment of a specific time that is non-negotiable, and structured into a daily schedule so that it does not have to be considered each day. No energy goes into scheduling, structuring, finding time, deciding whether to do it or not, weighing benefits and drawbacks. The time is reasonable and optimal, such as one hour. It's two o'clock, so you go to the gym.

You have an appointment with your doctor, your dentist, your child's teacher. You keep that appointment. You don't debate about whether you will or won't, bargain with yourself in some way by putting it off and saying you will do it next Tuesday. You don't feel virtuous if you do, it's just there, and you do it. An obligation. It requires no deliberation—just sticking to the plan. If that plan is to work out six days a week, then you stick to it.

In every sort of training, when you begin learning something new and see steady improvement, it is exciting and self-sustaining. Ultimately, when that improvement plateaus, it becomes natural to conclude that you have hit a limit, that you have achieved your maximum benefit. So, you stop forward movement and establish that plateau as a new normal. This is the reason people stop improving.

Our brains participate in this process. When something is new and exciting it stimulates our dopamine system, the reward chemical, so that we sustain efforts to continue that good feeling. Inevitably this startup system, the sprint system of dopamine, must transition to the marathon system mediated by other chemicals, chiefly norepinephrine. The experience of this marathon system becomes significantly less exciting and engaging. It often results in a disappointed, "Is that all there is?" This is a common experience for someone in therapy, coaching, mentoring. For the professional to understand this process as a natural brain phenomenon can help someone ladder expectations to guide sustained effort and longer-term results.

The Output Channel

What is the best way to teach and learn something new?

When you are explaining something or trying to remember information, first provide a context.

In a classic study three groups were given detailed verbal information, then tested for how many of the items they remembered after two minutes:

Group 1: given no context, remembered three items.

Group 2: given the simple context of "This information is about washing clothes," remembered six items.

Group 3: after listing what they remembered, they were then given the context that the items and actions were about washing clothes: their recollection was no better than the group without a context.

Group 2 did the best because they were given the context before the list of items and had a framework for organizing what they heard.

We construct a mental model—a schema—that helps us organize information into a story. A story helps us understand and remember.

Of the three types of learning strategies, which do you think yielded the best results:

- *Review of the material*
- *Test yourself*
- *Create a concept map to write the main ideas and relationship in a diagram*

Psychologists Jeffrey Karpicke and Janell Blunt found that the self-test of writing out the concepts outperformed every other kind of preparation.

This application of the output channel becomes an important component in all learning. A simple application is that a drill allows focus on a specific segment for attention and development. A drill can then isolate a weak segment for specific work.

Related research shows that to perform better, actual practice at retrieval of the material and enacting the skill are far superior to other methods. This approach is fundamental in sports as well as in academic, intellectual, and even artistic learning and performance.

Which reading method will result in the greatest testing success?

- *Reading eight pages of material four times in a row, trying to memorize it*
- *Reading the eight pages once, putting down the paper and writing a one-page summary*

Research shows that the second strategy of putting knowledge into action results in 50 percent greater success. Use of the output channel begins to wire the brain in a different way. To do the summary, you have to reflect, synthesize, and integrate the material to form it into a specific communication.

What will result in higher retention of written material: reading it with full concentration or reading it out loud?

A study at the University of Waterloo found that retention is 40 percent greater simply because of reading out loud rather than reading silently.

Learning effectiveness increases by using an output channel to summarize, outline, or apply what was studied. When an output channel is mobilized in the brain, it creates new neuronal networks and pathways to begin rewiring with the new information. The most immediate result becomes improved memory retrieval. Repeated findings by various investigators show that this type of targeted effort involving active reconstruction of what is learned can increase learning tenfold on average. In one study, when physicians' assistants requested that the patient write the date and time of the appointment rather than doing it themselves, it lessened the no-show rate by 18 percent.

Are there different output channel styles?

There are three distinct learning styles to focus learning: memorization, relation to what is already known, and self-monitoring.

1. Memorization
   A composite of studies by Jo Boaler (Stanford University) and Pablo Zoido (Organization for Economic Cooperation and Development) compiled results in several countries to determine that the lowest achievers in every country were the memorizers. Research has shown that emphasizing memorization, rote procedures, and speed impairs both learning and achievement.
2. Relation to what is known
   In various studies, groups learning passively by being provided with explanations perform only half as well as groups that proactively create their own resources and explanations. Generating information and processing explanations in an output channel complete a learning circuit in the brain, rather than only in a passive input channel. Additionally, actively integrating the new skill or new information with existing experience further creates effectiveness and mastery.
3. Self-monitoring
   Actively encoding information and practicing are enhanced by active monitoring.

Evidence-based practices show that greatest learning and performance occur with encouragement of a growth mindset in participants, emphasizing understanding and relatedness of material or skill along with its application. Whatever the type of performance, the key element requires using an output channel as close to the actual situation of performance or delivery as possible.

What kind of skill practices lead to the best long-term learning?

Some of the answers from performance and sports science help address this question.

Long-term learning can be maximized using three proven methods:

1. Space out practice schedules rather than compressing them into a short period.

   To train for a skill development, one training session each week for four weeks results in considerably greater skill acquisition than if all four hours are compressed into one time period. An example of several similar studies is of thirty-eight surgical residents who received four training sessions in a specific kind of microscopic surgery. Half received all the training in one day, the other half in one training session a week for four weeks. A month after training concluded, all the surgical residents were asked to perform surgery on a laboratory animal while experts who did not know about the experiment observed. The residents whose training had been blocked and spaced performed significantly better.

2. Deliberately challenge yourself.

Determine an area to work on, with specific attainable goals, over a specified period. Systematic and deliberate practice are required to get better at any complex skill, including to stretch current abilities.

3. Focus on each component separately but not exclusively for a sustained time.

Studying or practicing one component of information or a skill set is referred to as block practice. Doing one block and alternating with another block with deliberate practice shows greatest benefit.

How can you instantly access a developed practice skill?

Deconstruct the components and chunk the practice on each. An example is chunking the focus on the second tennis serve for an entire practice.

Bill Tilden, winner of a dozen Grand Slam singles events and ranked number one in the world for seven straight years illustrates: "My idea of intensive practice is to pick out one stroke and hammer away at that shot until it is completely mastered."

In developing their expertise, elite performers "chunk" information into operative, meaningful components based on effective patterns.

Studies that track eye movements of expert performers—pianists, athletes, surgeons, chess players—have found that with growing experience there is a faster and more seamless shift of selective attention to the clustering of information important to determining a next move. Mental representations and corresponding brain patterns develop. By contrast, although a novice may focus more consciously on the individual pieces or skills, those with expertise synthesize and integrate the relationship patterns into a seamless expression. The result is that elite performers respond more quickly and with less cumulative information and focus on crucial input more quickly than others. This chunking of information and brain process develops elite performance.

A wise coach or mentor adds value by collaboratively observing which patterns in creating automatic engrams work and which do not. And which work for specific circumstances or applications.

There is recent evidence that even when we do not intentionally practice something, we can passively absorb it. Showing an executive a successful negotiation of challenging factions and the synthesis of new solutions can effectively inform the observer. Observing how a skilled player executes movements and plays can help the athlete consider additional possibilities in their own execution of related moves. The best results stem from then actively putting the new scheme into action.

What mindset can best frame how you respond to stress?

The brain cannot tell the difference between excitement and anxiety. With the same brain activation for both, framing can determine subsequent performance. Framing an experience as excitement and challenge boots up a mindset to consider opportunity. Framing it instead as anxiety and threat focuses attention and energy on trying to calm down, manage stress, and overcome the experience rather than using it to boost efforts. Since the brain registers excitement and anxiety in the same way, the way you frame it determines the mindset of how you proceed. The Texas translation: It's better to ride a horse in the direction it's going.

A 2010 study found that those who view stress as facilitative have a 43 percent lower chance of premature death than those who view stress as destructive. Dr. Kelly McGonigal's book *The Upside of Stress* presents a large body of evidence showing that how we view stress significantly affects how we experience it.

To frame stress as an impediment to be avoided immediately affects performance. Viewing it as an essential readiness to engage and enhance performance creates a mindset to optimize everything that follows. Heightened physiological arousal then channels into enhanced performance.

Every performer experiences an energy activation before performance. Registering it as excitement to begin optimum engagement generates a mindset to actualize success. This awareness of experience and the immediate mindset framing initiates subsequent action. We choose how we respond to internal and external stimuli moment by moment.

Mindful self-awareness becomes a gateway to mindset selection. Mindset choice can then ideally frame performance for each task.

Decision Enhancement Tools

What will more likely motivate you to complete a task: focus on the small accomplishment achieved at the beginning or focus on the larger remaining work to be done?

Several studies have shown that the chances of success are increased in the early stages by focusing on the small amount of progress that has already been made rather than on the more significant amount that remains to be done. This focus creates a sense of effectiveness, and validation of successful progress.

Customer reward programs show how the built-in feedback mechanism of showing the progress made toward a free item or a flight upgrade results in significantly greater subscription and engagement in completion of the reward journey.

How can practice and performance be enhanced by better error management?

Mistakes, when handled constructively, have significant payoff in the development of deliberate practice, along with providing an opportunity for positive learning. Rather than a mistake or error being disruptive and eroding confidence, a composite of twenty-four studies in this area reveals two essential components:

- Focus on specifically what is to be learned
- Respond to an error by feedback without criticism or judgment

As with all deliberate practice, *how* a coach provides feedback can avoid perception as judgmental, critical, or pejorative. Positive examples include: "A mistake is a natural part of the learning process;" "The more errors you make, the more you'll learn;" or "You view an error as a highlight of what you can next learn."

A formal study of companies with a strong error management system and culture are four times more likely to be among the most profitable companies in their areas than those that have a weak error management system.

The DNA of Peak Performance: The Neurobiology of the Sweet Spot

How can the level of optimal arousal for learning and achievement be achieved?

The sweet spot is the place where the ball responds in the best possible way to the stroke of a baseball bat, golf club, or tennis racket. The sweet spot of peak performance is affected most by two psychological factors: self-regulation and focused attention. A continuum beginning with focused attention and interest can move to optimal arousal and optimal performance. Or it can be impaired because of anxiety or distraction. Optimal arousal is a crucial component of creating and sustaining a sweet spot.

Three neurochemicals combine to create the neurobiology of the sweet spot. How we get to the most productive and effective mental sweet spot in any performance, from life to business to athletics, can be learned and trained. Getting to that zone, applying the specific skills, and systematically improving and sustaining those efforts are all part of performance science.

The anatomy of arousal involves a balance of neurochemicals that make up the essence of peak performance.

- **D**opamine, the pleasure transmitter.

- **N**orepinephrine, the neurochemical regulating attention and alertness.
- **A**cetylcholine, the neurochemical most involved in the actual peak performance itself—released at a critical time of new learning and brain neuroplasticity with focus and optimum learning machinery turned on.

Dopamine

The neurotransmitter dopamine plays an essential role in motivation. We have typically understood its role as providing pleasurable reward for behaviors. Several animal studies suggest that it is more linked to wanting to pursue a given behavior, and its continuing release does not necessarily correlate to whether the experience is pleasurable or even liked. Neuroscientists now suggest that the brain uses dopamine to make predictions of how rewarding an experience will be. Dopamine levels are highest when an experience exceeds expectation, informing how much pleasure we derive. Dopamine asks, "Is this new or unexpected?" If the answer is perceived as a "yes," attention focuses, and new learning begins.

This means that rather than a way to spur behavior, the brain uses dopamine as a signal to predict what will provide reward. This function emphasizes that what we expect and what we get are encoded differently. This results in preferring a smaller reward now to a bigger one later, which neuroeconomists call delay discounting. It's harder to save for the future, because both future time and need are abstract terms, while current pleasure is the proximate experience. There is no brain pleasure chemical for long-term goals.

Norepinephrine

Norepinephrine enhances alertness to help us respond immediately to any threat as well as to regulate attention and alertness. We become alert to detecting errors when performing, and activation of norepinephrine is optimum when we feel challenged to perform a task better and error-free.

Acetylcholine

This neurochemical turns the brain on to be receptive to new information and to consistently establish new neuronal pathways of learning. Acetylcholine drives the learning machinery of the brain. We activate this chemical component by paying specific, conscious attention and engaging in physical as well as mental exercise, especially when we are exposed to new and important learning. In this way, acetylcholine parallels dopamine by sharpening focus.

What is the role of positive and negative feedback?

Everyone has threat and reward circuits. Rewards are intense but often short-lived, while a threat is not forgotten. Significant success performance can be derailed by a single remark that is perceived as negative.

Those who need predictability and certainty are most comfortable with rules and systems, often generating stress with deadlines and emergencies. This group may engineer extrinsic stimulation such as procrastinating or creating an artificial deadline. They may generate a last-minute flourish to finish a project. The extrinsic stimulation can create more focused performance by this group.

Those who perform better without requiring external stimulation for high performance practice and perform more independently of the external circumstance.

Reflections on these two styles may guide an optimal performance mindset and neurochemical balance. For example, if you focus on the things that you can determine and the environment where you may have most control, creating structure and deadlines may result in better performance.

How can self-awareness best be used to monitor practice and performance of sweet spots?

Self-awareness is essential in both deliberate practice and peak performance. This includes recognizing an optimum amount of stress as well as structure. What it takes to maintain an optimum and steady level of arousal is ideal to attain and maintain a sweet spot. Knowing your personal peak performance profile is crucial. Recognize situations in which you are:

- Optimally initially aroused
- Over-aroused

You can then attend to more advanced details—developing deliberate practice rituals in the process of excellence. Habits, in essence, form the foundation of deliberate practice and peak performance.

A habit simply means we have rewired our brain to not have to think about the behavior that has become a default mode, an automatic execution. The more that each skill becomes automatic, the greater the focus and energy can be on the next step. A basketball player knows how to dribble without thinking about it and can focus on performance flow.

Default habits are the result of deliberate practice as prelude to mastery and peak performance. Habit becomes incorporated into an identity, which makes it permanent in your mind and brain for automatic patterned repetitions. As habit becomes automatic and rewires to a default system, energy is freed to focus on the next habit to develop.

Practice Rituals and Habit Development

I like things you don't have to think about.
George Costanza

Professor Jerry Uelsmann at the University of Florida divided his students in film photography into two groups on the first day of class. The left half of the classroom would be the "quantity" group. They would be graded on the amount of work that they produced. On the last day of class, 100 photos would get an A, 90 photos a B, 80 photos a C. The right half of the room would be the "quality" group, graded only on the excellence of their work. They needed to produce one photo during the semester, and to get an A it had to be as perfect an image as possible.

At the end of the term, every one of the best photos were produced by the quantity group. These students throughout the semester took many photos, and experimented with composition, lighting, dark room methods, all the while learning from their mistakes and honing their skills. The quality group focused on the theories and ideas about perfection but had little to show for their efforts other than their theories and one mediocre photo.

The quantity group were continuously putting their ideas and skills into action, modifying the results, and proceeding organically.

Action is a behavior that will deliver an outcome.

To become routine and ultimately a habit, the steps must be simple, specific, frequent, and repeated. The sequence itself is best when it is easy, repeatable, and rewarding. A framework of a culture or community can add impetus and impact to repeated experiences. An external trigger as cue is ideal.

Who do you want to become?

- ☐ Align with your performance identity
- ☐ Achieve and sustain your sweet spot in each practice session

Develop a system:

- ☐ A pattern of the factors that influence your performance
- ☐ Structure work environment, hours, and tasks for optimum arousal to fit the situation
- ☐ Balance practice, performance, rest, recovery
- ☐ Awareness of biorhythms daily and weekly
- ☐ Determine which state to enter for each performance

To enhance arousal, consider specifically which of the neurochemicals of the DNA of peak performance need to be tweaked:

- If you feel unengaged or unmotivated, enhance dopamine with positive self-talk, humor, or some external change.
- For energy arousal, imagine something you may be afraid of, such as a missed deadline, to increase norepinephrine.
- If there is a natural downtime or slump during the day, enhance acetylcholine with a workout.

If arousal needs to be modulated or lowered, consider a brief mindfulness meditation, a period of unfocus of a walk in nature or other unfocused time for rejuvenation. For example, a break spent in nature can improve emotional regulation and create an antidote to stress.

These key points provide an overview of attaining and sustaining your sweet spot:

- Engage optimum arousal for the specific task.
- Have fun (dopamine release). My favorite grandmother, as you saw from the Dedication of this book, was a dopamine expert who repeatedly said, “If you’re not having fun, you’re not doing it right.”
- Focus attention on what’s important.
- Challenge your brain to release the optimum amount of norepinephrine.
- Know your biorhythms, preferences, and way of achieving arousal.
- Know the conditions for achieving and sustaining arousal.
- Structure your environment to fit your biorhythms and personal performance profile.

Framing Performance Mindsets

Brandon Webb, Navy SEAL sniper-turned-CEO, describes front sight focus as a state of intense concentration of attention and resources on a single targeted focus that blurs everything else in its specificity and intensity. While there is awareness of the entire context and everything going on in it, the exclusivity and intensity of attention directs to the one most important thing for full execution.

We each continuously talk to ourselves, whether we are conscious of it or not. We continually ask ourselves questions that will create, sustain, or disrupt an optimum performance state. Most of these questions and most of the self-talk is not conscious. You can self-talk your way into success or out of it. Peak performers exhibit complete and total confidence with self-talk that sustains and even enhances that peak state.

Exceptional performers have a systematic approach to the elements of deliberate practice and pay careful attention to each of the components in preparation. Then, in performance, they ignore that system and focus only on the flow state—the performance zone. Done right, it becomes a hardwired brain pattern. The key is entering that performance state of mind, staying in it to not pay attention to any of the components of its operation, and to not be distracted by anything external.

Sustaining flow is the baseball player not responding to being hit with a pitch to sustain focus, a Navy SEAL knowing when not to shoot, a CEO not reacting to a taunt at the annual meeting.

How can the way we frame a situation or endeavor make a difference in performance?

Dr. Jeremy Jamieson at the University of Rochester studied the impact of mindset framing on performance. He found that how people view stress can make it either beneficial or crippling. and processed.

College students preparing for the Graduate Record Examination (GRE), an entrance exam for PhD program admission, were invited to take a practice test. Saliva samples were collected to measure stress response. All the students knew that the study was designed to examine the physiological stress response and its effect on performance. Jameson gave half the students a brief presentation to frame their pre-exam anxiety in a positive way, as validation of activation and engagement in the task. The other half of the students got no such preparation.

The students who received the mindset framing of positive challenge and enhanced performance did significantly better. Additionally, in a post-test second saliva sample, the students who performed better had a higher level of sympathetic activation from stress. This reappraisal of pre-performance anxiety as excitement and opportunity coupled with a belief in enhanced performance significantly affected the actual performance.

Several studies replicated these findings with professional athletes, Green Berets, Marines, and Rangers. The evidence suggests that positive framing of stress leads to enhanced performance under pressure,

significantly more than relaxing as preparation for performance.

Researchers at Jacobs University in Bremen, Germany with physicians and experienced teachers showed that those who viewed their anxiety as helpful and beneficial were less drained and burned out by their work at the end of one year. They viewed their anxiety as the antithesis of depletion, leaving them to frame this experience as challenging, contributory work.

Anxiety framed as excitement fosters a belief and perception that contributes to enhanced performance of both mental and physical tasks.

Simply stated, if you view anxiety as a sign that you will do poorly, that will become true. If you view it as fuel for enhanced performance, that will become true. Long before brains were studied with the sophistication that we now know, Henry Ford put it simply: "If you believe you can, you're right. If you believe you can't, you're right."

What matters most is the cue of optimum performance coupled with the meaning that you have attached. When a signal of anxiety is interpreted as a prompt to initiate an optimum response, it ignites a performance story accessed in the mindset software developed by deliberate practice.

What interventions become negative prompts?

Telling someone who is anxious to calm down takes away the internal point of reference and belief in that individual to self-regulate and determine an optimum meaning. When someone is trusted to self-regulate and enter a zone of optimum performance, this trust helps that person rise to the challenge.

Organizing efforts to avoid or overcome emotional triggers that provoke anxiety will have the opposite effect. We engage what we avoid and reinforce what we pay attention to. As many of us know from raising adolescents, whatever behavior we respond to will either sustain or enhance its frequency. Good as well as bad.

Any stressful experience, from a major presentation to an important athletic competition to a future-determining exam, can benefit from this mindset framing to help focus, to interpret anxiety as performance energy, and to fulfill the challenge response.

This stress mindset intervention by a coach, mentor, or teacher has potential not just to change performance but to change lives.

This performance framing mindset not only enhances performance but also adds years to your life. The Framingham Heart Study, one of the longest-running epidemiological studies in the United States, shows that challenge response physiology enhances both cardiovascular and brain physiology and longevity. The brain rewiring based on mindset intervention benefits both resilience and performance.

When you feel challenged and frame it as active energy, it enhances confidence and fosters better performance. This has been shown to be as true in business negotiations as it is in championship competitions. Your response to pressure situations is determined by how you think about your ability to handle them.

Peak Performance Habit Development

We are what we repeatedly do. Excellence, then, is not an act, but a habit.
Aristotle

Our conscious minds have everything to do with setting up the framework and system of deliberate practice yet very little to do with the performance habit that is created.

The purpose of deliberate practice is to create performance habits that are done automatically without thinking about them. Habits are a bottom-up (System 1) processing that you do not decide to do each time you do them. A true habit is performed automatically, without conscious decision or planning.

Habits become most effective without conscious decision-making selection or monitoring. For example, I don't decide each day to go to the gym and look at my schedule to carve out time to execute that plan. It is a default mode, an automatic schedule and habit that I do each day at the same time without deciding and without thinking about it.

A habit is the greatest conservator of energy. As a foundation for mastery, habits apply energy to the next action step. Structure creates freedom, and habits conserve energy in that process.

Learning the basics, the fundamental principles of any practice or discipline, allows creative contributions to that process. A synthesis of various practices and disciplines creates a truly unique application.

A key to growth and transformation is incorporating self-reflection and redefinition as a component of that identity. The content must necessarily become the process:

- "I am an outstanding basketball player" transforms to "I am a lifetime athlete with mental toughness."
- "I am an outstanding CEO" becomes "I build and create new and evolving possibilities."

A focus on the system of change rather than on the goal builds identity-based habits, based on who we wish to become. Whatever change we generate in behavior, unless we also transform our identity—the fundamental operating system of who we are—we will return to that fundamental identity. To make a change permanent requires a transformation of identity to correspond with the new behavior.

We build a habit by repeating behavior enough times until it becomes automatic. With repetition, the brain rewires for this behavior to become the default mode, so automatic that it requires no conscious thought and little mental energy. A cue activates this cognitive script of behavior + identity to enter the performance success pattern.

What contract will you make with your future self?

Civilization advances by extending the number of operations we can perform without thinking about them.
Alfred North Whitehead

Ulysses, king of Ithaca and hero of the Trojan War, was on a protracted sea voyage after the war to go back to his home island of Ithaca. He had a rare opportunity ahead, in that his ship would pass the island where the beautiful sirens sang melodies so alluring that no one had been able to avoid their magnetic pull. When they lured the sailors and their ships toward them, the ships crash on the rocks, drowning all aboard.

Ulysses knew that like everyone else, when he heard the music, he wouldn't be unable to resist it. But he created a present plan to deal with his future self. In his present rational state, he ordered his men to lash him to the mast of the ship and not untie him no matter how much he begged or pleaded. He then had them fill their ears with beeswax so they could not be seduced by the voices of the Sirens. He made it clear to them that they were not to release him until the ship was well past the sirens, nor were they to take the beeswax out until then.

We are each free to make a Ulysses Contract, to create a plan for a future self, a pre-commitment. Someone breaking an alcohol addiction ensures that they are not exposed to alcohol. Someone saves for the future by having an automatic checking account withdrawal the first day of the month to be placed in a retirement fund. Both are good one-time decisions.

Why is it incredibly easy to repeat bad habits and so difficult to form good ones?

Habits are based on the two fundamental principles of human behavior, both hardwired in the brain: to avoid pain and to seek pleasure. Behaviors that are immediately rewarded will repeat; those with negative consequences will be avoided.

What is the greater pleasure if you proceed with what you need to do?

What is the greater pain if you decide not to proceed?

Whatever we choose to do is based on how we imagine we'll feel when we do it. At times this may be to prioritize a delayed reward rather than an immediate reward, the inverse of how our brains are wired. What we experience as an immediate reward repeats; what is immediately punished is avoided.

To establish any habit, we must immediately feel effective and successful in what we do. Shrinking the change to make the next step tangible, specific, and simple enhances the possibility of making an effective step.

Making any change specific, tangible, and measurable enhances the success and the experience of effectiveness to form a habit.

How can you assess habits in ways to continually enhance performance skills?

A habit—the rewiring of the brain—becomes the bedrock of the pursuit of practice rituals. A consideration in this process is that once a habit is formed, we get accustomed to the routine of needing to pay less attention to the process. This means that as we gain experience, a performance skill can decline. This process of skill development, refinement, and improvement needs to combine with a systematic approach for self-reflection and objective review.

Every habit developed from deliberate practice needs to include a way to assess and fine-tune the habit. A systematic self-reflection incorporates structured assessment to include the following:

- Scheduling an appointment with yourself for a brainstorming session on a monthly, quarterly, and yearly basis.
- Reviewing your plans and their effectiveness on a weekly, monthly, quarterly, and yearly basis.
- Periodically reviewing the results of those performance habits to determine what needs to be enhanced and what need to be changed.

Incorporate a practice of change and habit development into your evolving identity. The model of how and who you are needs to evolve and transform to parallel your behavior to make change permanent. When it becomes permanent in your mind (identity) and your brain (rewiring), patterned repetition rewires neuronal pathways and networks. Because these processes are so embedded, we need a systematic and scientific way to understand and assess them and to consider new experiences that can become new habits.

How can you best sustain high performance in the face of ever-increasing pressure and rapid change?

This question, restated: *What makes some individuals flourish under pressure while others fold?*

High performance may relate to cognitive capacity in academic settings, with physical talent in sports, and with emotional understanding in interpersonal interactions, but an exceptional performance pyramid in any context combines and integrates:

- Cognitive capacity
- Emotional intelligence
- Values and sense of purpose
- Physical stamina and conditioning.

These performance pyramid components address mind, body, emotions, and spirit.

Performance Cues

Pete Maravich, the elite all-pro basketball player, continued to wear the same outer pair of socks from high school throughout college and his entire pro career, without daring to wash them. He believed these socks were linked with excellent performance. And he became right.

Another example of a superstitious cue is when Michael Jordan wore extremely long Chicago Bulls uniforms to hide his "lucky" University of North Carolina Blues underneath for each game. This superstitious ritual ushered in an entire fashion statement for the long, baggy basketball shorts that has remained standard for all players.

A cue can boot up a particular mindset to enter a performance zone. A gesture for a wedding toast or keynote, an image by an actor about to go on stage, a quick head (Jack Nicklaus), a tongue click (Daniel Wolpert), or "I got this" (Laurie Hernandez). Indexing an entire set of skills and information with a simple gesture can cue an entire mindset with all its deliberate practice skills embodied. A brief ritual, gesture, or phrase serves this purpose. For some, listening to a song creates this ideal state within a few notes. Earlier discussion applied a cue to regulate states of mind in the Neural Conditioning Program.

A performance cue activates a sequence of behavior that, when repeated, becomes hardwired and automatic. This coupling with action becomes an effective performance trigger when it is a simple, quick physical gesture or word. Repetition encodes the word or gesture with the performance.

Researchers have found that performance cues generate certainty as well as attenuate anxiety through the predictability of an optimum response.

Whether the classroom, performance stage, playing field, or boardroom, high-stakes activities can generate stress-filled experiences and challenge peak performance. Finding the right technique and strategy to perform optimally in each specific situation becomes the challenge. Especially at times of significant stress, a focus on what to do generates better performance flow and results than a focus on how to do it. Even more specifically, focus on a keyword related to the outcome of an immediate performance generates the best results when performing under pressure. For example, professional and collegiate golfers focus on a single word that represents the motion such as “smooth” when putting, which generates better results than focus on words that represent technique such as grip or body position.

A one-word performance cue on the optimum action rather than technique or steps allows the default brain mechanisms formed in deliberate practice to operate without interference. This focus on outcome organizes brain pathways embedded through deliberate practice and activated by the cue at the time of performance. This cue of outcome focus directs the brain to automatically perform the practiced skill. When asked how to describe what they did after a superb performance, an athlete will likely not know how they did it or even be able to describe it. They have performed their best because they are not thinking about any step or performance, are not inside their own heads, and certainly not reflecting on what they’re doing while they’re doing it. Stopping to think, even for a second, about performance can disrupt the performance flow, detrimental to the outcome.

Psychologists Mike Anderson and Kristin Flegal asked both highly skilled and beginning golfers to take short putts on a flat green. One group then spent several minutes describing the putts they had taken, while the other group worked on an unrelated task. Then the golfers were asked to again perform the putts. The skilled golfers who described the past putts did significantly worse in completing their subsequent putts than those who had not tried to describe it and did something else instead. For beginning golfers, performance did not vary significantly between the two groups.

For well-practiced activities, thinking too much or focusing on the stepwise process of the performance can be detrimental. Sustaining the flow toward an outcome rather than the mechanics can avert mistakes.

A London woman I worked with in mentor coaching recognized that she spent a significant portion of her day in disconnected states prompted by her responses to other people, both personally and professionally. She used the Neural Conditioning Program to be aware of the emotional triggers that prompted the disconnections so that she could quickly recognize the process. She developed a mantra of touching a necklace medallion she'd bought for this purpose; it was always ready as a cue to prompt a focus phrase ("Now") and physiology (two deep breaths) to get grounded and centered so that she could move into an ideal state and behavior. Ultimately, simply touching the medallion instantly booted up her ideal state.

A gateway habit serves as a cue for an entire sequence of behavior that is designed to enhance both mindset and skill. The bedrock of any deliberate practice is the skill that is developed along with the corresponding new identity. You take informed action in small steps to confirm and solidify the person you want to be, the bedrock of your sense of self. This focus on the process, the system rather than the goal, emphasizes how the output channel of actions systematically shapes habits. Predetermined decisive moments systematically create the building of new habits. If you have a schedule of going to the gym six days a week at 2 p.m. and do that no matter what, it becomes a habit that takes no energy or debate about whether you will or won't, do or don't engage it. Like work, it's there; something seems missing if it isn't. You show up. Nothing interferes except perhaps family emergencies. In this way it becomes your identity. You have created a system to fill in various goals over time. The system is always there, no matter what, and makes good habits easy and bad habits hard.

A body in motion tends to stay in motion, and a body at rest tends to stay at rest. When a habit is established, it takes more effort to stop the habit than to continue it. Cognitive processing, decision-making, or any form of thinking about it presents an opportunity cost. Energy must be diverted to a different, cognitive part of the brain. Self-control and willpower become opportunity costs for the execution energy of a habit.

Do different types of cues work better for some people?

For performers whose primary representational style is auditory, a single word or phrase can immediately induce an optimum performance zone. I mentioned the all-pro cornerback who, after each play, would say to himself, "Reset." He knew that after every play, whether exceptionally good, bad, or even one that did not involve him, he needed to be grounded and centered in his performance zone for the next play. This works well for episodic sports such as football and gymnastics rather than for the sustained performance flow of sports like basketball or for executive functioning.

For kinesthetic organizers, a physical cue such as pressing the center of your palm and imagining that a signal travels to your brain to create calmness and quietness of your entire nervous system can be very effective. George Kittle, the all-pro tight end for the San

Francisco 49ers, touches the tattoo of the Joker on his wrist before each play as a performance cue.

For visual organizers, picturing a specific scene that is meaningful for both groundedness and peak performance becomes optimum.

What is a blueprint for forming an optimum performance habit?

Habits are automatic behaviors triggered by specific cues. Actions and ultimately habits can be systematically engineered. A behavior begins with a cue—a trigger that activates a sequence of behavior that, when repeated, becomes hardwired and automatic.

First is the cue, the internal or external spark to enter an optimum state of mind containing a practiced behavior, word, or gesture. After the cue comes the action, the preprogrammed behavior that is automatic response without deliberation and is synonymous with the ideal state of mind containing deliberate practice. Once entered, the state of flow becomes automatic to engage that state and the practiced behavior for optimum performance.

To sustain the performance flow, the cue may need to be repeated, either when distracted or regularly to sustain focus throughout the task. Or both.

At times for some individuals, focus on a single key word related to the outcome of the performance provides the necessary focus to sustain immersion in the performance flow state. One-word cues focus on the result, such as saying "smooth" while executing a golf putt. The basketball player may simply use the word net when shooting a free throw. The single word not only boots up the entire performance mindset but also activates the visual image of the successful result.

When the cue is an action or gesture, you may be better able to remember, as memory is grounded in the body. Each time you practice any sequence, such as a mantra, begin with the physical cue to initiate the sequence. This sequence is a complete circuit in your brain when it goes through the output channel activated by the action step of performing the cue. For example, dribbling the basketball twice while saying a focus phrase and taking a deep breath in for relaxation and breathing out to release any tension; practicing a wedding toast by picking up a wine glass. A simple gesture initiates an entire performance mindset and behavior.

What other factors can serve as performance cues to frame mindsets?

We've learned a great deal about what influences the learning brain to enhance both optimum learning and performance, whether academic, intellectual, or artistic. A composite of research (Thad Polk's The Learning Brain) shows four factors that play a crucial role in performance:

1. Self-Efficacy

Jane Elliott, the originator of Workplace Diversity Training and one of the thirty most notable educators of all time according to WHO (along with Confucius, Plato, and Booker T. Washington), once served as an expert content contributor for my MasterMind group and presented the results of her famous "Blue eyes—Brown eyes" exercise for her class the day after Martin Luther King Jr. was assassinated. Her exercise illustrated how people will live into the expectations others have of them. The exercise, conducted with her third-grade school class of eight-year-olds, designated the blue-eyed children as the superior group, giving them extra privileges and access to playground equipment, including extra recess time. She would not allow the brown-eyed and blue-eyed children to drink from the same water fountain and emphasized differences between the two groups by singling out students, using negative aspects of the brown-eyed children to emphasize a point. The next week she reversed the exercise, making the brown-eyed children superior. The compositions that the children then wrote about their experience created a resurgence of awareness of the effects of racist behaviors on performance and regard. Her work was the forerunner of diversity training and the need for enhanced awareness for optimum performance in various arenas.

Self-efficacy has a tremendous impact on learning, first by determining what people will attempt to learn. When you believe you are capable of learning something, you try; when you don't believe you are capable, you may not try. For example, a bad experience in math or negative feedback can contribute to a lowered sense of efficacy in math, resulting in perhaps not trying to learn. If someone believes they will not learn well, this often becomes a self-fulfilling prophecy determined by their effort and commitment. They may either not try or choose a less risky alternative that produces a compromise. The degree of self-efficacy often determines the amount of persistence at a task.

An application of this process has been demonstrated in studies of gender and racial bias in learning to show that when the expectations by a mentor or teacher lower expectations and, therefore, the student's performance. The tyranny of low expectations is well-known from studies of white racial framing.

2. Perceived Control

When people visit a physician and the physician prescribes a medication, just over 50 percent of people do not fill the prescription. Of those who do fill it, just over 50 percent fail to take the medication as prescribed. So of those who are perhaps worried, go to the trouble of making an appointment, driving to the physician's office, and going through an examination or questioning or both, less than 25 percent follow through and take this expert's advice. They were instructed, given a directive and an order, but it did not become their story. The antithesis of this model of "compliance" is collaboratively co-creating a new story together with the patient/client/colleague/protégé as point of reference to incorporate autonomy, competence, and connectedness to self and others.

When you develop your own story, it minimizes the need to comply or perform in a dictated way. When you own your story, you own your performance. We most engage what we help create.

Perceived control is the perception of how much you believe you determine what you do, as opposed to perceiving that external forces outside your control determine what you do—the exam was unfair, the referees were biased, the unlevel playing field is sloped against you. If you don't believe that how you practice and how much you work will significantly affect your outcome, why bother?

Those who believe they can do better engage a growth mindset of deliberate practice to improve, which determines a far different outcome. Perceived control is related to several growth mindset variables, including motivation, sustained effort, degree of engagement, and less boredom. Those with higher perceived efficacy perform better in several dimensions, from physical to academic.

3. Effectiveness and Mastery

Two factors determine successful completion of a goal more than any others: challenge and attainability. A goal should be sufficiently challenging to engage full effort, combined with knowing that attainability is possible to feel effective and experience mastery. Setting goals, either for oneself or collaboratively with a coach, can be most effective when they are specific, measurable, attainable, relevant, and time-bound: SMART goals.

Some studies have shown that when goals are set at a high-low range rather than a fixed number, that participants more likely attain the goal within that range. An example would be to lose between one to two pounds per week for 20 weeks, rather than setting a goal of losing 1.5 pounds per week, and more effective than setting a goal of a 20-pound loss.

4. Perceived Value/Purpose

Meb Keflezighi in 2014 became the first American to win the Boston Marathon in over thirty years. His win occurred one year after the terrorist bombing at the 2013 race. Keflezighi credits his performance to inspiration he felt for those who died in the terrorist attack the year before. He wrote their names on his race bib so that he would run with greater purpose and motivation. "Toward the end I was remembering the victims who passed away," he said, "They helped carry me through."

The value placed on what is being learned contributes significantly to successful learning. We must care about what we learn as well as have it fit with our own ideals of meaning and purpose. The highest perceived value is that which aligns with our own identity.

Purpose can become an orienting perspective to serve as a magnetic pull registered by an internal compass. When your purpose is for something greater for yourself or for others, this enhances the likelihood of pushing on.

When we have a greater purpose for why we do what we do, such as to enhance the lives of others, to be a catalyst for achievement and fulfillment, it makes daily annoyances tolerable, perhaps not even engaged.

In her book Grit, Angela Duckworth emphasizes that grit is a hallmark of high achievers in every domain. Gritty people hang in and persevere when others quit. Dr. Duckworth found that grit is not innate but can be cultivated over time. While there is no single way to develop grit, the trait is often accompanied by a strong sense of purpose. Especially when the going gets tough, gritty people draw upon a greater cause for inspiration and stick-to-itness. As Duckworth and her colleagues wrote in a 2014 paper, "Highly aversive experiences may become more bearable when they are viewed as having positive consequences that transcend the self."

Are there stages to creative mastery?

Mastery involves self-awareness and self-regulation, two key components of emotional intelligence and optimum performance. A significant aspect of mastery is accessing the optimum brain state for a particular task. Examples include being in a creative, expansive state for writing and in a focused, attentive state for editing.

Creativity is a whole-brain experience, right and left, top and bottom webs of connections. To be centered and grounded is to have access to an entire range of states of mind, to be in an optimum position to synthesize and integrate information from various sources located in different regions of the brain.

The four stages of creative mastery are:

1. Define and frame the creative challenge.
2. Focus on specific ideas and information regarding the identified task.
3. Relax and center to fully engage in a performance flow.
4. Execute the task with focused, sustained engagement and implementation

The basis for self-mastery is a combination of awareness and integration of internal states to then enter the precise state matched to the task. This process will be systematically applied in the deliberate practice components that follow.

Chapter 5. Deliberate Practice Strategies

A simulation is an opportunity to practice but frequently it's also a wake-up call: we really don't know exactly what we're doing and we had better figure it out before we're facing this situation.
An Astronaut's Guide to Life on Earth, Chris Hadfield

Richard A. Clarke served as national coordinator for security, infrastructure protection, and counterterrorism under four presidents: Reagan, Bush, Clinton and Bush. He engaged in a specific form of deliberate practice as head of cybersecurity for the U.S. government. At a small gathering of cybersecurity heads of Fortune 500 companies where I did a Master Class, he described how he trains agency executives and chiefs of operation for national emergencies. His crisis training consists of repeated three-hour stress tests that he calls "war games," which simulate practice for various scenarios of cybersecurity hacking. He and his team fully simulate attack scenarios so that every conceivable option will be considered and practiced for an emergency.

He emphasized that the war games cover "everything that could happen" so that each person practices repeatedly and under stress to know how to do it in case of an emergency situation. He described how the simulations of disaster make each participant uncomfortable and how they learn to master it. When they make the right decision, "We increase the stress so they would know how to handle variations of the worst scenarios." The simulations occur over seven to ten days with progressive practice on disaster scenarios. These hypothetical exercises at the highest level of government apply the fundamental principles of deliberate practice for national and international security.

Each of the heads of agencies involved in the 9/11 attack had done everything that happened during that attack in simulated war games every three months for the previous several years as directed by Clarke. He emphasized that the results of 9/11 were circumscribed and mitigated because the scenarios had been covered in the stress test practices. Each person involved knew how to respond because they had responded to each facet of a similar simulated disaster a number of times in the war games.

This elite form of deliberate practice has saved countless lives because of his expert execution.

The key element is effective, focused practice in the sweet spot—that centered, attuned zone in which you can immediately know if there is any slight mistake. Every skill is a form of memory, and deep practice develops that skill.

Deliberate Practice: An Overview

Are you getting better at the things you most care about? Or are you not improving much at things that matter to you despite spending a lot of time working hard at them?

Consulting with Professor Anders Ericsson, Dr. Angela Duckworth indicated that she had been jogging an hour a day, several days a week, since she was eighteen years old but had not gotten faster in all that time. For thousands of hours, she was doing the same thing repeatedly.

Dr. Ericsson, who has spent his professional lifetime studying how experts become experts and what they do to practice and perform exceptionally, asked Duckworth the following questions:

1. Do you have a specific goal for your training?
2. Before you go for a run, do you have a target in terms of the pace you would like to keep?
3. Do you have a distance goal for each run?
4. Is there a specific aspect of your running you try to improve each time?
5. What do you think about while you are running?
6. Do you have a coach?

After she answered each question with a “no,” he concluded, “I think I understand. You aren’t improving because you’re not doing deliberate practice.”

The prevailing theory for decades held that experience was the key to expertise. The more someone practiced, the more expert they became. Ten thousand hours to develop significant expertise. Yet compelling research shows that we don’t gain expertise from experience alone.

How you practice informs how you perform. The repeated admonition of my favorite coach: “Practice like you’ll play.” Most of the learning and growing occurs during practice, not during performance. Intense focus on crafting a specific goal with openness to input from a coach provides significantly more benefit than massive repetition or even regular practice.

Ericsson and his team found that the number of years of practice had no correlation with how successful a clinical psychologist was with patients. In several instances, experts such as physics professors and practicing physicians did not do as well as newcomers in their respective areas. Repetition of the same experiences is different from deliberate practice focused on improving.

Older and more experienced physicians paradoxically often perform worse than younger, less experienced colleagues. The reason for this documented finding is initially not obvious. While the younger physicians have undergone more recent training and attained more current knowledge in school, the continuing education of experienced physicians should bridge that gap, and the gap should be further widened by years of experience in the trenches. But this is not the case.

With artists, intellectuals, and athletes, neither experience nor practice is the crucial variable. The primary determinant of superior performance is deliberate practice. Expertise comes not from the total number of hours of practice, as in the ten-thousand-hour rule, but from the type of practice that fills those hours. Ericsson demonstrated that deliberate practice could take many forms of cumulative experience, including "formal education, private instruction, coaching or mentoring, exposure to domain-specific role models, and various forms of self-education."

In fact, practice itself can make you worse. Every shot that misses makes your aim worse. The creation of muscle memory is a process of myelination and of rewiring brain neuropathways. Repetition of specific intended motor skills rewires so that each time, over and over, it becomes faster, easier, and smoother. The drawback is that a skill performed in the wrong way can become hardwired. Deliberate practice confronts the myth that it only takes effort to improve, that repeatedly trying harder will result in getting better. If you are not improving, it does not mean that you lack basic talent but that you may not be practicing in the best way.

The solution is not to try harder but to try differently. For example, to approach a barrier from a different direction, such as by working with a coach—someone who's familiar with the obstacles and can suggest ways to overcome them. Ericsson emphasized how deliberate practice is much a more significant factor of success than are physical attributes. Further research by his team and those he inspired, including me, have resulted in a more developed system, structure, and application of his groundbreaking work in deliberate practice.

Deliberate Practice: The System

Deliberate practice is a prototype for a habit-forming scientific technology of behavior. Performance behavior needs continuous evaluation of the results so that it can be revised as needed for improvement.

Practice deliberately. Evaluate results. Modify continuously. Develop a performance habit.

The science of deliberate practice sets it apart from repetition. The following nine components generate elite performance in business, sports, and arts:

1. Engage the optimum state of mind for a specific practice segment.

The characteristics of elite performers in business, sports, and various individual achievements are all similar, and all start with mindset. Belief in potential, capacity, and improved performance consistently becomes the mindset to overcome prevailing myths of limitation, plateaued performance, or fixed ability and talent. It involves, as well, transcending the belief that you're designed to get better at something if you do it consistently.

Fully focus each practice segment. Ericsson and his team found the necessary component to be "engaging with full concentration in a special activity to improve performance." Deliberate practice involves structure and focus with clear goals and feedback. It requires attention specifically to engaging the performance state of mind directed to each specific practice task, and each segment in the overall skill development.

2. Establish a well-defined, specific goal to improve on—not just "getting better."

Purposeful practice relies on the fact that the human brain and body respond to challenges by developing new abilities and new neural pathways to neuronal networks.

Five questions to ask for each performance goal:

- Is your goal specific?
- Is your goal measurable?
- Is your goal positive?

- ☐ Is your goal inspiring to you?
- ☐ Is your goal displayed?

In performance psychology, three types of goals are important: *outcome* (to define the specific result), *performance* (goals that focus on performance relative to how you have done before), and *process* (how you perform a specific skill set). The right kind of practice carried out over a sufficient period leads to improvement and expertise.

3. Determine your purpose.

Deliberate practice also requires a reason to keep at it, a purpose. Deliberate practice is not immediately or inherently pleasurable, so a strong sense of purpose is necessary to sustain efforts. A sense of purpose can fuel the brain and body to respond to challenges and develop new abilities with new neural pathways and networks.

A consistent pattern emerges: regular training results in changes to those parts of the brain that mediate the functions required and are challenged by the training. Only the right kind of practice, carried out over a sufficient period, leads to improvement. Deliberate practice is significantly more important for peak performance than predefined ability or talent.

People who have become experts acknowledge that the thousands of hours that they put into intense deliberate practice with full concentration is not always fun but is a means to the end of improving their performance. While the innate pleasure is of effectiveness, they are willing to pay the price even when they don't feel like it. Some players rebound from defeat by briefly reviewing mistakes and what can be learned, then focusing on the specific steps to the next success.

4. Determine a challenge beyond your comfort zone.

   Doing the same thing over and over without a focused stepwise plan for improvement may not result in getting any better.

   The basic principle of any kind of practice: if you don't push yourself beyond your comfort zone, you will not improve. Ten thousand hours of practice can be doing the same thing ten thousand times or systematically extending each practice segment just beyond a comfort zone.

5. Establish a time structure.

   Deliberate practice requires optimum structure and use of time, as it can be sustained only for a limited time each day. More frequent, shorter sessions, each lasting eighty to ninety minutes with half hour breaks in between, seem to be more productive than longer practices.

   Up to four hours a day makes optimum use of available mental and physical resources for effortful practice. Sustaining concentration for deliberate practice limits the number of hours but optimizes their productivity.

6. Visualize the successful completion of specific goals.

   Jack Nicklaus stated the essence of deliberate practice in his own model of visualization: "I never hit a shot, even in practice, without having a very sharp, in-focus picture of it in my head. It's like a color movie. First, I 'see' the ball where I want it to finish, nice and white and sitting up high on the bright green grass. Then the scene quickly changes, and I 'see' the ball going there; its path, trajectory, and shape, even its behavior on landing."

7. Review what works and what does not, with a central goal of consistent improvement.

   The 10,000-hour rule applies to a complex task, characterized by development of pattern recognition and sophisticated motor responses. However, other aspects of expert decision-making are not automatic and intuitive even after expertise is hardwired. Certain situations require cognitive reflection and logical thinking about choice and action, situations such as those faced by first responders, military commanders, and elite athletes.

   One of my favorite writers, Geneen Roth, was an expert content contributor in one of my MasterMind groups, and in response to a question about writing her bestselling books, she revealed that she never lets any writing be seen until she's done at least thirty edits. Each edit improves, refines, and focuses the writing and incorporates expert feedback.

8. Use feedback from a coach to gauge when you are doing something right and how to specifically improve.

To explore talent and its myth, several depth studies of child prodigies were conducted and found that those who seemed to be an exception were instead testaments to deliberate practice. For example, in Genius Explained, Michael Howe found that Mozart had accumulated, with mentoring and intensive training by his father, at least thirty-five hundred hours of practice by the time he was five years old. Gifted performers with similar stories about intense early exposure include Tiger Woods, the Williams sisters, David Beckham, and the chess-playing Polgár sisters.

As a six-year-old chess prodigy, Josh Waitzkin, author of The Art of Learning, articulated the principle of focus: "I learned quickly that when I thought about the people watching, I played badly." Josh's chess coach would ask him when he made an important decision to explain his thought process. They then collaboratively explored other ways of thinking, playing, understanding an opponent, considering different operations. This description of an elite coaching process began with a six-year-old boy as protégé. Waitzkin describes this process succinctly: "A heartfelt, empathetically present, incrementally inspiring mom or dad or coach can liberate an ambitious child to take the world by the horns."

Feedback from an expert coach needs to be immediate and on a specific aspect of performance.

In-the-moment advice on how to progress should lead to concrete improvement in performance.

And then later we take over that function and responsibility ourselves to create an internally motivated and balanced experience.

9. Develop self-correcting mental representations of the evolving skill in deliberate practice to permanently etch its operation and to incorporate it as identity.

The central purpose of deliberate practice is to develop mental representations that organize the execution of skills. The process then becomes a self-identity. Recognition of each practice success step validates the achievement to incorporate into a performance identity.

Deliberate practice is designed to improve and hardwire those representations over time. The characteristics of elite performers in business, sports, and other endeavors are all similar and involves this fundamental process.

What is the best structure for a deliberate practice segment?

Certain practice structures have been shown to be more effective to enhance skill development:

1. Research all related information and best practices.
2. Determine specific practice activities, including mental and physical components.
3. Schedule a time and structure for specific components.

4. Practice deliberately, beginning with an optimum mindset, focused attention, and sustained energy devoted to the specific task for a practice time segment.
5. Complete a drill of focusing on specific—often the weakest—points of performance.
6. Spend a portion of time on retrieval and the output channel, putting into practice the specific skills addressed.
7. Review and reflect on the arousal state and intensity of the practice session to see if any adjustments need to be made.
8. Get feedback from an expert coach to immediately use in practice revision.
9. Create a structure or procedure to immediately retain both practice and feedback information.
10. Integrate the new stretch practice immediately to push the edge of a comfort zone. Revise the concept to relate it to what you already know.
11. Ask: Did I try something new and extend beyond my previous practice and experience?
12. Review your results and, after a brief pause, integrate the new practice you learned with what you already knew.
13. Decide what needs focus for the next deliberate practice session.
14. Decide what aspects of the new practice need to be further addressed systematically to extend the skill.
15. Determine what additional information is needed to plan and structure future segments of deliberate practice.

Deliberate Practice: The Applications

Where can deliberate practice be applied?

850 undergraduate students learning physics were divided into three sections of physics instruction by researchers at the University of British Columbia, including a Nobel Prize winner in physics. One section had the usual teaching with lectures, weekly homework, and tutorial sessions. The other two sections, equally matched for ability, had parallel traditional instruction for eleven weeks. Then one of these two latter sections continued traditional teaching methods, the other applied deliberate practice, including exercises and engaged discussion of questions and challenges. They created answers, discussed them, and got immediate feedback on their problem solving. They were additionally offered thoughts to ponder about particularly difficult areas.

The average score of students in the traditional section was 41%, while the average in the deliberate practice class was 74%. The students in the deliberate practice group got more than two and a half times as many right answers as those in the other section.

Deliberate practice establishes specific, well-defined goals, and a conscious knowledge of exactly what you want to accomplish with every repetition. The repetitions are informed by expert information and ongoing feedback. Practice does not make perfect; practice makes permanent. Only perfect practice creates perfect performance. Practice of a slightly incorrect skill sequence will result in permanent etching of that incorrect sequence. Only purposeful deliberate practice will result in enhanced expertise and skill development.

Imaging studies demonstrate how the brain adapts and grows in response to specific informed repetitions of skill development. Deliberate practice modifies the structure and function of the brain, increasing the ability to perform skillfully.

Deliberate practice is difficult, relentless, repetitive work over a long period of time. The two "child prodigy" musicians I worked with took fourteen and seventeen years, respectively, to gain international recognition in their fields. The Olympic gymnasts I have worked with took a similar period of time, also with near-exclusive dedication to their skill. Their practice was very specific to their signature skill. A somewhat longer period of dedicated practice may be necessary for writers and professional athletes. Common to each of those I have worked with was relentless dedication combined with a growth mindset and the use of a series of specialty coaches as their skills evolved.

Also common to each were countless hours of repetitive practice, exclusive focus on specific performance skills, and relentless dedication despite occasional boredom and lack of fun. Their coaches often used exposure to and collaboration with role models combined with growth mindset practices.

The same framework, although in a different context and with different application, applies to successful executives and practicing professionals. Each is an artist, whether business or professional. Each learns the best things to do, consistently enhances skills by learning to do them right, and always practices and grows with a mindset of being "the best." For each, it is a passion as well as a purpose with commitment.

Is there an optimum state of mind for each deliberate practice segment?

Depending on context and circumstances at a given time, we act like different people. This is simply a phenomenon of different states of mind. One study of this, by Dan Ariely and George Lowenstein, pioneers in studying behavioral economics, found that physiological arousal created a different and enhanced performance. The brain works differently depending on the state of arousal, and the "hot state" can create a unique mindset and software system that can elicit quite different responses in performance depending on the state of arousal.

One takeaway from their study is that deliberate practice must include practicing in various arousal states—a continuum within a given performance range. Competitive arousal is itself a continuum that has various degrees and levels of active engagement. Competitive arousal leads to increased blood flow in the anterior cingulate cortex and the anterior temporal cortex, regions of the brain involved in emotionally related processes. When the blood flow to these areas is increased, there is decreased blood flow to the regions of the brain that receive and integrate sensory and motor signals related to higher level thought, judgment, and expression.

The arousal fueled by competition must be considered and practiced as surely as any individual skill. The brain has a number of pathways, and the degree of arousal will lead to the automatic, unconscious choices of pathway, so this specific deliberate practice must include the ones that work best for different situations, circumstances, and skills. Unless practiced, arousal can short-circuit a usual pathway and lead to diversions, underperformance, and chokes. Arousal can also make us take unnecessary risk unless this arousal is also practiced and developed in performance situations.

One example of deliberate practice with specific stressful application is our penchant for action bias. Faced with uncertainty or ambiguity, especially when in the context of stress, we naturally tend to do something rather than nothing, even if it is counterproductive. We want to act in order to feel effective rather than experience the ineffectiveness of "passivity." This is a common phenomenon in investing when the market moves significantly up or down; the tendency is to do something in response rather than nothing. In sports, it may be to rush the pass or the shot rather than to engage a contemplative pause that may introduce a better choice. A physician who is unsure of a diagnosis may prescribe something or call it a virus to bring closure.

Is there a brain-friendly way to give more effective feedback to a player?

A recent Gallup survey found that 26 percent of employees agreed that the feedback they get improves their work. That's pretty low.

The amygdala in the midbrain scans at all times to determine if a message has a social threat component. If it perceives threat, it instantly and unconsciously moves to a defensive, protective position and derails the impact of the actual suggestion.

Great feedback usually does two things. First, by asking a question, it lets the player's brain know that feedback is coming. It also engages the player to collaboratively explore a possibility and engage a buy-in by also looking at the question. This buy-in is the essence of autonomy, the choice of being effective in exploration rather than simply being a recipient of information or criticism.

The feedback formula continues when the feedback message is wrapped in with another question: “How do you see it?” Or “What are your thoughts about this?” This makes for a collaborative conversation and joint problem-solving rather than feedback that can too easily be perceived as critical, pejorative, and unilateral.

Feedback can be a regular component of every conversation; you don’t have to wait for it.

In deliberate practice, feedback is best when it is immediate, before repetition grooves a bad habit. Instructive, informed, and observed practice is essential in honing elite performance. The development of a working alliance between the coach and player is the most valuable framework in any kind of conveyance of skill development and learning.

Practice with immediate feedback and correction improves performance, while more experience without it can make you worse. Openness and the flexibility of using feedback constructively leads to improvement.

Are there specific qualities of an ideal coach and player?

Gerard Roche surveyed 1,250 successful executives to find that two-thirds had a coach. Those who did made more money and were happier in their careers than their peers. Roche found that on average these executives made 28.8 percent more in income and received 65.9 more in bonuses. Research by Shane Snow finds that entrepreneurs with coaches raise on average seven times as much money for their businesses, and experience three and a half times as much growth. Coaches also shrink the time it takes for someone to reach expert level, along with enhancing their performance.

Many accomplished performers have no idea how to pass their skill and expertise on by teaching. It is important for the coach to have skill and experience in teaching, not only in performing.

A related aspect for the player is being coachable, being open to input, lessons, and especially self-reflection based on that input. Input and ideas can potentially come from anyone at any level, not just experts and seasoned coaches. The key is a player's readiness to receive and use instruction and feedback. Growth evolves from how we handle change.

Is innate talent, dedicated practice, or superhuman effort what explains some remarkable athletic and intellectual feats?

The fastest softball pitch is 67 mph.

Softball pitcher Jennie Finch was a gold medal winner in the 2004 Olympics, who challenged the best pitchers in professional baseball to hit her pitches. Major league baseball hitters are accustomed to hitting 95 mile per hour fastballs, and the softball is bigger.

Albert Pujols, the greatest hitter in a generation, was the first of these. Other outstanding hitters followed including Brian Giles, Mike Piazza, and Barry Bonds.

They all struck out. In fact, only one hitter managed to barely touch one ball—a small tip for a foul.

What accounts for the best batters in the history of baseball not being able to hit a softball pitcher with a ball coming at them 30 miles per hour slower than their accustomed smaller baseball?

Same question, different context.

Both grandmaster and novice chess players were shown an entire chessboard with difference configurations of pieces. In five seconds, a grandmaster chess player could recreate from memory an entire board. A novice could only reproduce about 50% of the chessboard configurations, after viewing them for 15 minutes. And, when both expert and novice players were given a random assortment of chess pieces – configurations that would never appear in a real game – both expert and amateur performed equally. Why?

There are no engrained performance patterns in the brains of those who have not developed these mental representations in deliberate practice. Even if related patterns are well-honed, such as baseball and softball batting, there is no cross-over.

Expert baseball players can predict the pattern of the ball as soon as they see the release from the pitcher's hand. The pattern and position provide the information needed to determine whether to swing at the ball or not, because the initiation of the swing needs to begin just after the ball leaves the pitcher's hand. When Jenny Finch faced Albert Pujols – at the time the best batter in the history of baseball – Pujols had no database of brain pattern development to anticipate what would happen when the softballs were released. Everything about the trajectory and patterns of the softball was different than the baseball, where he developed his expertise.

Likewise, the grandmasters remembered “chunks” of pattern configurations and instantly identified the variations of patterns they had encoded over deliberate practice time in their brain wiring. Chess masters see a familiar order and structure, whereas the novice is overwhelmed by the randomness and the massiveness of non-patterned and thus disorganized information.

With sustained, deliberate practice, you can reach and then extend your potential and your initial goal, to make possible what was not even considered previously.

The system of deliberate practice encodes the entire skill set operation into an evolving mental representation. The mental representations organize the performance sequence, as well as solidifies your identity as a performer. This evolution and transformation of identity is what makes change – as well as performance flow – permanent and automatic. Without it, you will immediately revert to your previous behavior, the hardwired default mode. The new patterns of performance, referred to by neuroscientists as "chunks," become mental representations in long-term memory.

The growing ability to recognize and incorporate meaningful patterns in deliberate practice develops skill become automatic, a part of performance flow.

These mental representations allow a chess master, quarterback, executive, or farmer to glance at a situation to recognize patterns to get an immediate sense of what to do next, without having to think about it or process it consciously.

The Role and Importance of Belief

The key to achieving is looking at the ultimate goal. It's believing, and then focusing completely on the next step in front of you.
Julian Edelman, Relentless

A young boy once imagined being an athlete and being part of a team. For him, any team would do. But he couldn't even make the church baseball team, because he couldn't throw from third base to home without the ball hitting the ground. He was cut from his junior high basketball team. He turned to smoking by the sixth grade and boosted fresh pies from a delivery truck that stopped at the bowling alley where he hung out.

There was one sport left that he could attempt in junior high. He tried out for the ninth-grade track team even though he had attempted in previous years without success. His run in the 400-meters lasted about 200 meters, and he did not make the team.

In tenth grade, he heard the cross-country coach speak at an assembly. "Many of you boys have done poorly in junior high sports, but don't be discouraged. Everyone grows at a different rate, and some of you still have plenty of growing to do."

This statement gave him a renewed belief in possibility, and in his first cross-country race, he placed twenty-first in his school, placing him on the C team.

This young man persisted. On a team bus trip, his coach, Bob Timmons, privately asked him how fast he thought he could get in the mile. Ten years earlier, this coach had seen Roger Bannister run a mile in under four minutes. Timmons told this young man that he could become the first high school runner to run a mile in under four minutes.

He ended the first track season with a 4:08 mile. He followed that by training like a professional, running a hundred miles in a week. In his junior year, Jim Ryun ran the mile in 3:59 to become a national sensation. That summer, on the 1964 U.S. Olympic Team as a nineteen-year-old freshman at the University of Kansas, he set a world record time in the mile of 3:51.3.

The coach who believed in him had seen Ryun's potential to live into that belief. ESPN later ranked Ryun ahead of Tiger Woods and LeBron James as the Greatest American High School Athlete of All Time. His coach had simply planted a seed of belief.

A related body of research shows the importance of hope combined with deliberate practice. Hope provides a dynamic motivational system for the learner. Sibling to belief, hope propels sustained commitment to practicing and achieving performance goals. Charles Snyder and colleagues have even found a way to measure hope and developed the "Hope Scale." Hope, like belief, is consistently related to positive outcomes due to persistence of goals and the belief that multiple positive outcomes can be found or created. Fueled by hope, someone continues to seek alternative pathways for reaching their goals. This practically means that we continually come up with different ideas about how to get there.

Hope, self-efficacy (the belief that you can master something), and optimism are all component expectations that contribute to goal attainment. When the three were measured, hope trumped as the foremost predictor of independent success.

Beliefs are the personal software that drive behaviors. A belief is something we have concluded and continue to assume, not necessarily derived from logic. Not all beliefs are conscious. We pick beliefs that appeal to us and anchor those beliefs in other assumptions we already hold. We don't notice contradictory ideas and often dismiss them when they don't fit the existing belief.

Beliefs collectively form a coherent identity, to make experience consistent with expectation. Changing a belief is tantamount to changing an increment of identity.

When evidence changes, we don't automatically change our minds. In fact, we change our minds only very slowly, and only in those instances where we have to. Experience generates more vivid memories than any information that we passively read or hear.

When expert opinion conflicts with our core belief and identity, we tend to discredit the expert. We not only hang on to preexisting beliefs but may also shop for additional or even maverick experts to confirm our beliefs.

The Role of Discipline

Champions keep playing until they get it right.
Billie Jean King, winner of thirty-nine Grand Slam titles in singles, doubles, and mixed doubles

Discipline requires patience in the process of developing skills. Patience with each component and the synthesis and integration of those skills combine into a working practice that becomes the default mode. This involves at times tolerating the frustration of focusing on what does not feel comfortable, on what you most need to work on, and the persistence to continue even though practice is frustrating. Trying something new when you don't know how it will turn out requires a belief that it will ultimately improve your performance. Tolerating times of feeling lost, clumsy, or confused at the initiation of a new practice or skill set. Recognizing that expertise in one area does not immediately transfer laterally to expertise in another area. Exceptional performance means consistently and patiently working on the process to the highest level of physical and intellectual endeavors.

Patience and discipline apply to every aspect of preparation and performance. Impatience may seek a shortcut, force an outcome, push a faster result, look at what might have been, compare to someone with a more accomplished performance, or lose a performance state of mind to a temporary frustration. The performer labeled by Tennis Magazine as one of the ten greatest players and "the game's greatest overachiever," Ivan Lendal said, "I'm going to do it until I get it right, and I'm going to keep doing it and doing it for hours and hours and years and years."

Patience requires belief that you will be better and achieve an optimum performance by loyally engaging the process to get there.

Discipline has been described as a three-step process:

1. Determine specifically what you want.
2. Decide exactly the price you must pay.
3. Choose if you are willing to commit and pay the price.

Discipline combines work ethic with performance ethic. The framework is a belief system in success, a purpose for everything that you do.

Ninety-five percent of those who lose weight on a diet regain it, with most gaining back a bit more than they lost. Ninety percent of all startups, New Year's resolutions, and post-heart attack resolutions fail. The focus is on the goal, the promise, rather than the system. Changing any habit or creating a new one requires focus on the system: having a plan and the discipline to stick to it. Rather than focusing on the outcome, focus on the process, the system of creating the outcome.

Amazon founder and CEO Jeff Bezos in his commencement speech to Princeton University's graduating class captured how our lives become the story of our choices. He emphasized that when we are at the end of our lives and sharing our story, "The telling that will be most compact and meaningful will be the series of choices you have made. In the end, we are our choices."

Learning Zone and Performance Zone

We have two performance-related mindsets: a learning zone and a performance zone.

In a learning zone, the goal is to improve, to concentrate on what you want to master, to expect to make mistakes, and to learn from them. The learning zone maximizes growth for future performance. Deliberate practice occurs in the learning zone rather than in the performance zone.

Learning zone characteristics include:

1. The goal to improve
2. Focusing on what you want to master
3. Expecting to make mistakes and learn from them

Deliberate practice etches an informed default pattern by repetition, correction, and further repetition. Deliberate practice ingrains new motor as well as cognitive skills to bring about mastery and to make it automatic. Deliberate practice always involves having a skilled observer who can offer feedback.

In the learning zone, there are four simple steps to change behavior:

1. Identify the goals.
2. Determine the mindset and behaviors required to achieve them.
3. Develop an action plan.
4. Program a new identity to incorporate the changes.

With developed skill, the entire performance zone process becomes a procedural memory, done without thinking or observation. Thinking about the process of skill execution becomes part of a learning mindset, not a performance mindset.

In a performance zone, the goal is to do something as well as possible, to execute. A learning mindset focuses on mechanical adjustments and refining technique. Performance mindset relies on kinetic memory and performance flow of execution. Effective performers do not focus on the workings or mechanics of their muscles, but practice to rely on kinetic memory. We use memory to forget, which frees performance energy.

In a performance zone, goals include:

1. Entering a performance zone mindset to access the skills of deliberate practice
2. Maximizing immediate performance
3. Executing in the best way possible while sustaining the mindset

For a practiced skill, beginners can benefit from thinking more, but experts can be distracted from flow by thinking more. An example of this phenomenon is a tennis match in which a lesser player compliments an opponent on a brilliant shot and then asks, "Wow! How did you do that? Did you shift your grip or adjust your elbow a bit to do it?" The player asking the question has made her opponent think consciously about a usually unconscious mechanism. This slight shift—even when the better player does not answer but nonetheless hears the question—is enough to disrupt a smooth, automatic flow pattern and generate slight change. The imperceptible shift from automatic, well-practiced unconscious flow from the Bottom-Up System is disrupted by engaging the Top-Down System.

How can you enhance your experience in the learning zone?

The answer is the entire spectrum of deliberate practice principles and applications. The people who continue to engage in the learning zone continue to improve.

Columbia psychologist Dr. Jennifer Mangels studied the brains of people with fixed mindsets and people with growth mindsets. When those with fixed mindsets received feedback, the brain dwelled on negative feedback, overshadowing accompanying corrective suggestions. Those with growth mindsets took in the corrective information and performed much better on a second test. They believed they could improve and did.

The shift to a growth mindset, in which one takes in information and uses it for enhanced performance rather than self-critical shutdown, becomes a crucial component of the learning zone and its purposeful practice.

The foundation of the learning zone is an innate curiosity that leads someone to curate advice and co-construct learning.

Framing a learning zone to develop expertise includes these components:

1. Believe and understand that you can improve—a growth mindset.
2. Want to improve a particular skill, with a specific purpose of each practice session.
3. Have an idea/plan about how to improve, what to do to improve, and how to use deliberate practice.

4. Consider the learning zone as a low-stakes situation, and expect mistakes, with a purpose of improving.

If players think that a mistake will make others think less of them, they may feel stressed and not take the risks necessary for learning. On the contrary, if they believe that mistakes inform learning, curiosity and exploration result.

1. Create practice spaces where mistakes are accepted, are to be learned from, and can be addressed by a coach with feedback.
2. Reflect on execution and performance about what could be done better. Observation, reflection, and adjustment occur in a learning zone.
3. Create openness by sharing what you want to get better at; ask questions about what you don't know; solicit feedback from others. Explore, ask, and listen for what you are working to improve.

In deliberate practice, feedback is consistently necessary. Without regular feedback, both body and brain lose track of their own performance and cannot objectively assess results.

Cognitive science research repeatedly demonstrates that specific feedback is superior to general feedback and that feedback on the last action performed is superior to feedback on tasks performed earlier in the day. Feedback provides reference points for your brain to guide behavior sequences.

Ask questions that are solution-based rather than problem-based:

- What can I do to make this happen?
- What can I create that will be exciting and engaging?
- What can I do to successfully navigate this impasse?

How can you enhance your experience in the performance zone?

Chris Sajnog trains Navy SEALs, arguably the best-trained athletes and warriors in the world. He has written best sellers including Navy SEAL Shooting, on how to prepare SEAL teams for battle. His statement “Start by training the most effective weapon you have: your mind. Your mind controls your body” is a summary of brain performance training. He uses the SEAL acronym to summarize the initial mindset components:

Sit down,
Eyes closed,
And
Listen to your breath.

The purpose of this brief mindfulness exercise is to get you immediately grounded so you can focus on the task at hand. The immediate quieting of the mind before a performance—for a SEAL, this is pulling the trigger—becomes the essential foundation.

Sajnog offers a strategy known as “GPS” for this focused training:

Gather intelligence: accumulate information to base decisions
Plan your route: a game plan of informed decisions

Start training: make the process an automatic default mode of flow

Common to practice and performance is maintaining focus and flow, with practice to return to this state again and again. Performance in this flow state seems effortless. The reset, to immediately reenter the performance zone and mindset of deliberate practice-based skill execution, is essential and distinguishes champions perhaps more than anything else within the performance zone.

What does the performance of chess players, rock climbers, artists, surgeons, Italian performers, Navajo sheep herders, and Chicago assembly line workers have in common?

Their peak performances were studied to show that the optimum results were greatest in the flow states. And produced the greatest enjoyment.

Flow, a total immersion in an activity so that "...nothing else seems to matter. The ego falls away. Time flies. Every action, movement, and thought follows inevitably from the previous one, like playing jazz. Your whole being is involved, and you are using your skills to the utmost." (Mihaly Csikszentmihalyi)

A summary of the value of creating a system for practice and performance is from George Bartzokis, M.D., a UCLA neurologist said, "All skills, all language, all music, all movements, are made of living circuits, and all circuits grow according to certain rules."

That structure of a system of practice has been shown to be the bedrock of the best performers in the world whether artists, athletes, pilots, bank robbers, or chess players. It is how a penniless Russian tennis club with only one in-door court has created more top 20 women tennis players than the entire United States.

What is the best way to minimize stress in various experiences?

The answer, from analyzing a decade and a half of studies reviewed by Stanford psychologists, Geoffrey Cohen and David Sherman found two significant, powerful results. When someone connects with their values, it helps them see the meaning in their lives. When people have their values in mind, they not only are more resilient to stress, but their individual effort and support of others increases. Adversity is temporary, a setback is something to overcome, rather than a self-definition. Cohen and Sherman refer to these findings as a "narrative of personal adequacy." It is not the stress experience itself, but what you tell yourself about it that determines a successful response. When viewed as consistent with a personal identity of ideals and values, responses become consistent with that identity. If you stumble temporarily, revert to that core identity.

The most powerful force of the human psyche is that identity, and any behavior that is not seen as consistent with core identity will eventually be abandoned. Any behavior that is not incorporated into a transformation of a basic internal model of identity will not last. That behavior which is incorporated into identity becomes permanent. Deliberate practice becomes the neural engineering of skill enhancement as well as identity.

How does establishing a goal set up performance success?

A goal does not distinguish a winner from a loser, or success from failure. There is nothing magical about a goal. What distinguishes success from non-success is a system of small stepwise improvements that lead to a specific outcome. The system and the goal are both important.

While goals may set a direction, the system needs to be a specific and proven focused, stepwise strategy for success. When you want to change, focus on the system. A system of strategic and continuous stepwise improvements leads to a successful outcome. Problems are solved at the system level, not the goal level. The system refines, improves, and addresses a growth process that will determine progress and then goal achievement. The system is the map.

Two challenges in changing any behavior:

- The mind is inclined to create certainty by repetition of the known outcome. This is a bias to want immediate closure and predictability (even if it's not the result you want).
- The brain has hardwired repeated behavior and has an error detection mechanism that alerts to anything other than repetition of the familiar.

Research on the deliberate practice mindset shows that anyone can improve with the right approach. If you're not improving, it does not mean that you lack basic talent, but it may be because you are not practicing in the best way.

What can we learn from the most successful performers about a structure for each practice?

Dutch psychologist Adriaan de Groot was one of the first to systematically study the difference between good and great. His initial research with chess players has since been replicated in other performance areas. Simply put, we can increase our working memory and performance expertise by grouping things together: chunking. Chunking helps us store more information and make better decisions. These chunks accumulate and allow the performer to recognize patterns more quickly and effectively in various situations.

The art and science of deliberate practice has four components: chunking, repeating, correcting, and mentoring.

1. Chunk the entire task.
   The chunk looks at a skill to develop as a whole task to understand the scope and breadth of the task, of what it will look and feel like, to see it clearly and fully illuminated. The chunk is the megacircuit that will be developed. An example would be to chunk a practice segment on the first serve in practice.

2. Deconstruct the components and proceed one step at a time.
   Any skill is made up of its component pieces or circuits done one at a time, in a progressive synthesized way that leads to larger groupings of new interconnected circuits. The purpose of deconstructing is to understand the individual components, to see those that most apply, and to put them together in a planned sequential way to repeat.

3. Apply slow, focused development.
   Football coach Tom Martinez puts this aspect most succinctly: “It’s not how fast you can do it. It’s how slow you can do it correctly.”
   Slow it down to learn the stepwise construction, the architecture, before speeding it up to a normal execution.

Understanding the individual distinct components, the small steps, allows you to focus on the specific, precise component of skill. Initially doing this slowly allows you to recognize errors quickly to correct them.

To see yourself executing the skill is the ultimate in visualization. When repeated sufficiently, the visualization rewires the brain to create the experience that is being imagined. This big-picture vision is composed of individual stepwise segments: sensory input from each of the five senses; the picture of individual motor skills activated in coordinated fashion; and the mindset of successful achievement, including thoughts, feelings, and cognition associated with that success.

Peak Performance Practice Plan Summary

1. Define a purpose and objectives for a task and for each practice.
   - Begin each practice with a focus on the purpose and the objectives for that segment of time.
   - Focus and sustain engagement in the state of mind in which that skill was practiced.
   - Remove any distractions to focus only on the task at hand.
   - Do only one thing at a time, the specific focused practice task.

2. Manage States of Mind

- Develop a self-awareness to enter a state of mind specific to a practice and performance task.
- Develop a method to instantly engage that state, such as a performance cue, focus, and physiology.
- Manage this state to sustain the engagement of a flow experience to access and sustain peak experience.

3. Establish systematic goals and a stepwise process of reaching them.

- Establish a goal for each practice task that is a just-manageable challenge, one that barely exceeds your current developed skill.
- Keep the next challenge just a bit out of reach but attainable.
- Remember to stay totally focused and regulate states of mind within each segment of deliberate practice.

4. Establish blocks of practice of fifty to ninety minutes, with rest and recovery in between.

- If a task is new, start with a smaller amount of time, even as little as fifteen to twenty minutes.
- For all deliberate practice, the maximum limit for each segment should be a two-hour working block.

5. Revisit and review the framework of a growth mindset throughout each practice.

- Reframe any anxiety as excitement and opportunity.
- Practice gratitude for the stress and challenge that are steppingstones to improvement.
- Reframe stress as a natural physical way your body prepares for a challenge.

6. Build in segments of rest and recovery framed as part of practice and preparation.

- Practice mindfulness meditation as a method of mental and physical restoration
- Recognize positive self-talk and the benefit of positive, brief, focused conversations with yourself.

7. During the breaks between practice, step away from the task and engage a relaxing focus, such as a walk in nature or meditation.

- Learn to listen to physical and mental needs.
- Recognize moments of insight and allow your unconscious the opportunity to un-focus periodically.

8. Remember that good and adequate sleep is a part of both practice and performance.

9. In a deliberate practice routine, develop a method of instantly entering a performance state and sustaining that state. These may be two related though different internal methods.

- Incorporate in a warm-up routine, for whatever type of performance it is, a mantra for immediately engaging an optimum state of mind.
- Have a specific cue or routine linked to optimum performance behavior.
- Practice the cue and routine as deliberately as the skill itself.
- Be sure the cue and/or routine can be done anywhere anytime, instantly, effectively, and consistently.
- Determine how you devote energy and brain power to by making the positive and beneficial aspects automatic.
- Match practice and activity with energy levels.

• Consistently structure and schedule every part of your day to become automatic.
• Recognize your biorhythms, the time of the day you have the most and least energy, and plan tasks accordingly.

10. Recognize the importance of social context.
• Surround yourself with positive people and consistent support.
• Establish a culture of performance, with everything and everyone supporting that purpose.
• Recognize what to keep, let go, avoid, and enhance.

11. Beliefs drive behavior. Behavior drives performance.
• Remember to show up consistently and predictably.
• Act. Evaluate. Adjust. Proceed.

12. Develop and sustain a focus on a purpose greater than yourself, the reason for doing and being.
• Recognize and integrate activities consistent with that purpose.
• Align needs and ideals with strategy and goals.
• To sustain motivation, create a map that specifies where you are and where you want to go so you can measure progress along the way, and immediately determine detour and distraction.
• Giving back and doing for others prevents burnout and enhances internal reward.

Chapter 6. Neuroassociative Conditioning for Optimum Performance

Neural Conditioning Program

When Southern Utah University's new basketball coach Roger Reid arrived, his team ranked 217th in free-throw percentage, lowest in their division nationwide. During practice, Reid had his players develop a mantra before each free shot, a three- or four-word phrase coupled with a deep breath for relaxation. He gave the example of “relaxed and smooth” when stepping up to the free-throw line but emphasized that each player needed to determine his own mantra.

Additionally, he simulated game conditions by abruptly stopping a player in practice and asking him to shoot two free throws. Reid simulated the mindset of pressure in a game situation by suddenly stopping to shoot a free throw. If the player made the shot, he got to take a breather. If he missed, he had to sprint around the court.

In two years, the team was ranked number one in their division nationally.

The Neural Conditioning Program offers a systematic way to rewire optimal performance behavior.

What you associate with a stimulus determines your behavior. To change your behavior, change your neural association. Thinking positively is not enough. You can think positively for a moment, but then you go back to what has already been established in the neuronal networks and connections of your brain. The effect would be the same as if you tried to change a software program by booting it up and talking positively to your computer.

Neural Conditioning to Make Changes That Last

!

Old Story		New Story	
Emotional Trigger →	Usual Response/ Behavior →	Mantra: Cue/Focus/Physiology →	Ideal Response/Behavior
!	!	!	!

Column 1: Emotional Triggers

An emotional trigger can be simply a word, gesture, object, or thought that cues an immediate state change that is then experienced as automatic and intrusive. Each state of mind consists of a pattern of neural firing of certain behaviors, feelings, and memories characteristic of that state. Each state is much like a software program on a computer and can be instantly activated by an emotional trigger.

Column 2: Usual Behavior (Altered-State Time Capsule)

Certain emotional triggers have the impact of creating an instantaneous reactive state change to immediately reenter the time capsule of an earlier state. Immediately upon entry, everything is the same as when that time capsule was first experienced—all the feelings, associations, ways of looking at things, anxieties, dangers, frustration, hopelessness and negative self-talk. The state change takes only a nanosecond.

When this occurs, the usual response is to try to figure out how to deal with a situation; to get someone to respond in a different way; to believe that expressing feelings will detoxify the experience; to think that creating a better solution this time around will be the answer. Of course, none of these work.

This process of instant response to an emotional trigger can result in a disruption of performance flow—a choke.

Column 3: Mantra: Cue, Focus, Physiology

The three parts of a mantra:

- Cue: a personal gesture or word
- Focus phrase: such as "Relaxed and powerful."
- Physiology: breathe in relaxation, breathe out tension

Mantras can be used in various situations to regulate states of mind, especially about emotional triggers that can instantly change a state of mind. Professional athletes and actors use it to get grounded and centered for their performance.

A summary of practice including a mantra:

- Develop a mantra: cue, focus, and physiology. Mantras can calm and keep you from overthinking in a high-pressure situation. A mantra is designed to interrupt an automatic response to an emotional trigger and reroute it to the optimum behavior.
- Focus on the target, not your mechanics. When you bowl, think about aiming for an arrow on the lane rather than your approach. When firing a gun, focus on a clear sight rather than your trigger pull. Barbara saw herself breathing calmly and simply observing the family gestures and words that had previously been triggers.
- Don't slow down. Slowing down allows you time to think about it, which will derail procedural memory flow.
- Practice under pressure. When you practice under the same conditions you'll face when you must

perform, you establish the mindset that you will enter in the actual practice.

Column 4: Ideal Response

What is the ideal current behavior in the context of the emotional trigger?

Recognize the emotional trigger so that you can use a mantra to instantly get grounded and move to the preplanned ideal response (Column 4).

Each of these changes can be immediate mindset transitions with a strategy to recognize the emotional trigger to reboot a state of mind to engage a planned ideal response.

The lateral movement across these four steps systematically rewires emotionally altered states of mind and their triggers. The altered state is simply not activated when focus is on the mantra to get grounded and centered. It is much like when you get up to move and your lap is no longer there—it's just a memory.

The Four-Column Process Overview

In summary, focus on the emotional trigger and usual response (Columns 1 and 2) allows you to immediately recognize an emotionally based cue and the resultant state change. Cuing your radar to recognize both trigger and response as quickly as possible allows you to see the process of the state change rather than staying stuck in the content of the altered state. Like a time capsule, that content will never change. You can't think, reason, feel, figure, or therapize your way out of a state of mind. That content will always remain intact, yet you do not have to inhabit that state. You recognize it as quickly as possible to get grounded and centered and then move into an ideal state (Column 3) and engage the preplanned behavior (Column 4).

Moving horizontally across all four columns requires focus and systematic attention. As you do this repeatedly, you will notice that repetition of the mantra will automatically induce a grounded and centered state. Because this neural conditioning ultimately rewires your brain using an automatic cue to induce a grounded state, you ultimately won't have to do the focus phrase and physiology each time.

Then, as you repeatedly move through all four steps to the ideal response, this will rewire your brain to couple the original emotional trigger with a now-ideal response. With consistent repetition of the new sequence, the emotional trigger that previously resulted in an instantaneous state change rewires the brain for an automatic ideal response.

The Neuroscience of Lasting Change

How do you condition yourself to make changes that last?

Victor Frankel was a Jewish psychiatrist in a Nazi concentration camp during World War II. While death was certain, he observed that about one out of every twenty-five of his fellow prisoners somehow managed to survive. He set about studying the characteristics of those who survived and found that it was what the survivors focused on that made the difference in their survival.

While twenty-four out of every twenty-five focused on their pain and inevitable death, those who survived created meaning—a purpose—for their suffering rather than accepting their fate and wondering why God was allowing them to die. For example, they constructed a reason to survive so that they could tell their story to their children, to make certain that this kind of atrocity would never happen again. It turned their suffering into something that would make a difference, a purpose that provided a will to live.

What you link inside your head—the meaning that you give—determines your behavior. You can change your behavior when you change the meaning. You can reprogram your associations and rewire your brain.

When you change the meaning of an association (neural conditioning), you change your behavior. There are three key principles of neural conditioning:

1. Identifying the cues/triggers for the behavior.

   The meaning you attach to a trigger determines your behavior. Observe the cues (usually emotional) that trigger an automatic behavior pattern.

   Questions to ask:

   o What are the cues or triggers for the automatic behavior pattern?

   o How can you interrupt your own pattern once you have identified it?

2. Recognizing what to change.

   The first two questions for bringing about any change are:

- What is it that you want to change?
- How would you measure that change?

The question of what you want to change initiates an assessment of how much you recognize authorship of your story and how much you own it. To recognize and own a story is essential to changing it.

The entry point may, however, may be the third step of assessment: How is that working for you? To acknowledge that what you're doing isn't working may be the initial step to systematically change your plan.

Belief and behavior questions may illuminate what people say as well as what they do, especially if there is a discrepancy. For example, after a declaration of what someone wants, ask, "What behavior would we observe that would clearly indicate that that's what you want?"

You must get to the point where you feel that you must change something, that you must change it now, and that you can change it. Believe that change will ultimately bring pleasure. Recognize that not changing would be ultimately more painful than the immediate pain of the change process.

Questions to ask:

- If you don't change your pattern, what will be the consequences?
- What is the pain associated with the current choice?

- What pleasure will result from changing?

3. Create a new association that empowers you.

   Condition a new empowering association with the same cue. For example, if you have limited yourself or feel stuck as far as making more money, link making money with strength, power, and possibility.

   Questions to ask:
   - What is the new association with the familiar cue?
   - What is the specific change you want to bring about?
   - What is the first step today you can take to get some traction?
   - What will you gain and enjoy with the change?

The science of success is the neuroscience of neural conditioning—of reprogramming your mind to attach meanings to what you see that will generate success.

Exercise: Transform threat stress into challenge performance

Awareness: Notice any signs of stress in a challenging situation, such as heart-pounding, breath-quickening.

Framing: This is your body's response to give you more energy.

Awareness: Notice any tension in your body.

Framing: This is your body's response to allow you to access your strength.

Awareness: Notice any other physiological responses such as sweaty palms or stomach butterflies.

Framing: These are signs of the task's importance.

Awareness: Persistence of tension

Framing: This activation is the embodiment of energy and strength.

Awareness: Negative self-talk or limiting belief

Framing: Convert self-talk into a positive, planned mantra. "I got this." "No matter what."

The Anatomy of Flow

How do you enter a mindset of total focus on a performance task?

In his book Flow: The Psychology of Optimal Experience, psychologist Mihaly Csikszentmihalyi describes the psychology of flow as "being completely involved in an activity for its own sake. The ego falls away. Time flies. Every action, movement, and thought follows inevitably from the previous one, like playing jazz. Your whole being is involved, and you're using your skills to the utmost."

Csikszentmihalyi found that the top creative and intellectual performers in the world shared three characteristics:

- Immersion of focus in a sustained state of flow
- Incubation periods of rest and recovery with practice and performance
- Self-reflection and self-evaluation of themselves and their performance

The bedrock of flow is accessing the state of mind of optimal performance for a task and sustaining the immersion in that state. In the state of mind of flow, the skills of your mind are directed and channeled into seamless execution. While entering this flow state, optimum performance results. Disruptions occur with any distraction, any focus on trying too hard, or observing oneself.

A flow state—being in the Zone—has a specific brain biological signature. Characteristics shared by many in this state include being fully and completely focused on the present moment, having a sense of time slowing down, intuiting how the next step will unfold, having a sense of connection with everyone involved, expanded consciousness, and enhanced performance levels.

Pleasure is the emotional marker for flow, and when we are absorbed in something and getting better at it, it simply feels good. This is effectance pleasure, the immediate experience of mastery. This pleasure at being effective is the most basic motivation we have as human beings. The experience of effectiveness is a central motivating force of deliberate practice and excellent performance with resulting pleasure and mastery.

The Zone experience is one of optimal performance not only in sports but in any area of functioning, including executive and parenting. This state of flow directs and channels skills and creativity in the present moment to generate highest possible performance.

Revisiting Performance Flow

When the risks are big, it's where I feel most alive. In a weird way, it's almost a meditative thing. When there's a lot on the line, whether it's a big business deal or surfing a scary wave, I get so focused. Things slow down. The tiniest of details become alive, the feeling of a pebble beneath your shoe on a rock wall or the real meaning of a sentence in a business deal.

John Winsor, quoted by Jonathan Fields

How can you best sustain the performance flow?

Tim Grover described the total focus of his client Michael Jordan: "If one thing separated Michael from every other player, it was his stunning ability to block out everything and everyone else. Nothing got to him; he was ice. No matter what else was going on—the crowds, the media, the death of his father—when he stepped onto that basketball court, he was able to shut out everything except his mission to attack and conquer."

The primary characteristic of getting into the flow of a performance zone is an immersion in the process of the performance itself, not thinking about it. The process of sustaining flow may be enhanced by:

- Frame a positive focus for both the performance and the outcome
- Use a key word, gesture, or internal snapshot to create and sustain focus throughout the process of performance

- Don't slow down or think about controlling your performance
- Practice under pressure to simulate the entire experience, including mindset of the actual performance
- Focus on the goal, not the mechanics

Focusing on anything other than the performance execution can result in compromise or even a choke. Self-doubt, negative self-talk, or worrying about a situation and its consequences can derail the flow state and its performance. If you think about what may go wrong, you are likely to ensure it.

Activities best performed outside conscious awareness need to be framed in ways to create and sustain this flow state and performance.

> *Exercise: Managing Distractions and Disruptions to Sustain Flow*
>
> The Rule of Three: The human mind can engage essentially three chunks of information in short-term working memory. When more items are added, attention and retention decrease.
>
> Distraction: Something that interferes with or diverts full attention and focus.
>
> Distractions can be filtered by focus and flow. Disruptions need an active filter and a plan for how to respond. Distractions can be inhibited or redirected from irrelevant information to allow greater focus and synchrony of brain function.

A specific part of the brain, the middle frontal gyrus, filters distractions when trained. Dr. Srini Pillay distinguishes between proactive filtering of distractions and reactive filtering"

- *Proactive filtering*: Predicting distractions and knowing how to handle them when they occur.
- *Reactive responses*: Flexibly dealing with unexpected distractions to continue the flow of a task.

Disruption*:* An interruption of focus to cause diversion, with an accompanying mindset shift with the derailed flow.

A priority: determine a time and place where you will have no interruptions. In my home office, a service person knocking on the door is an interruption, so I do not schedule any service people or external appointments during my virtual work time with clients or training sessions. I even have the front doorbell disconnected and no call interruption on the telephone. During videoconferencing, landline and cell phone ringers are silenced.

Chapter 7. ROADMAP System for Performing Under Pressure

The ROADMAP System informs active listening and understanding of performance story components. The specific structure and strategy guide the strategy for improved performance.

The seven steps represented by the acronym *ROADMAP* introduce a systematic way for to recognize, own, assess, decide what to change, map changes, author new story lines, and then program new identity to incorporate the changes.

New experiences with as-yet-undetermined outcomes are inherently coupled with uncertainty, trepidation, and anxiety. To change performance, focus on the system. Doing anything new or different—achieving change in any manner—is a venture into the unknown.

ROADMAP States of Mind

With Integration of the Neural Conditioning Program

Any emotional trigger can create an instantaneous state change. An awareness of the process allows the ability to regulate and choose your response to any triggering event, internal or external. The key is recognition of the emotional trigger of the instantaneous state change (Column 1 of the Neural Conditioning Program) and the content of the altered state (Column 2 of the Neural Conditioning Program).

A specific feeling can trigger a state change, although it may be initiated by an external event. Other people and events may trigger unwanted thoughts and unpleasant feelings, but they do not cause them. The mechanics of how you respond are largely unconscious, stemming from the beliefs and automatic couplings in your mind and brain.

But you can become consciously aware; you can direct your choices. Self-awareness is the first step in transforming your thoughts and feelings and thereby your state of mind—the specific choice of software program you operate on.

You can use the ROADMAP System to develop awareness of feelings and their connection to thoughts and how both relate to the choices you make. The ROADMAP System® is simply a means of editing stories to redirect narratives for changes in behavior.

Exercise

Return to the Neural Conditioning Program. Work with the first emotional trigger you wrote. Go through these seven steps to demonstrate how to ROADMAP a state of mind for performing under pressure.

Recognize the emotional trigger that cues a particular feeling or automatic behavior.

> Recognize each emotional trigger that prompts a state-of-mind change (Column 1 of Neural Conditioning Program) to boot up a specific mindset. Cuing your radar to recognize an emotional trigger and the subsequent instantaneous state change allows you to

objectively and quickly recognize the process to become grounded and centered (Column 3) and move into an ideal response (Column 4).

Observe and own your present awareness.

Ownership and accountability are prerequisites of change. Recognize the state contents of any altered state (the beliefs, doubts, anxiety, negative thoughts, and self-talk of Column 2). Mindfulness of your story is necessary to change.

In the instantaneous imperceptible shift to an altered state, focus becomes directed to the content of that state, including beliefs, doubts, anxiety, negative self-talk, and recurring negative thoughts.

Own present awareness to refocus on the process itself: use a mantra to self-regulate rather than becoming stuck in the contents of the altered state time capsule.

Assess your emotions and feelings.

The automatic behavior results from the emotional trigger. Be aware of all feelings and sensations in your body. Be aware of what you are experiencing at this moment, and what you were feeling, even in a brief, signal way, that served as a trigger to change your state of mind.

If the feeling is anger, look at the assumption that caused the anger. Did you assume that someone needed to respond exactly as you wanted, as an extension of your desire, in order for you to feel happy? If so, the result would be ineffectiveness, and anger would be the counter to feeling helpless. Rather than management of anger, the assumption itself needs addressing.

Decide to engage in a predetermined strategy.

Establish a fully present, grounded state using a mantra—the three-part sequence of cue, focus, and physiology (Column 3 of the Neural Conditioning Chart).

Map an ideal response.

Plan an optimum response and behavior (Column 4 of the Neural Conditioning Chart). Instead of the emotional trigger coupled with the usual automatic response, create an ideal response for that trigger, a response to employ after regulating your state of mind.

Author new experiences.

Complete the behavior that is ideal, with the thoughts and feelings that match this new response. Recognize the feelings and internal conversation that become part of the ideal response.

Program a new identity.

Recognize that you have choices, that past behaviors do not define an identity. Incorporate this new model into your present identity. The mastery and confidence of effectively making informed choices evolve an identity of a growth mindset.

For each trigger and usual reaction (Columns 1 and 2), plan the ideal behavior in Column 4. The idea is to recognize the triggers and the reactive behavior as early as possible, rather than well into the unfolding of its cycle from inside the altered state. Plan the ideal behavior or response so that you can consciously substitute it. With repetition of this new behavior pattern, you ultimately groove it as a default mode without having to think about it. With repetition, the original cue is rewired to the ideal behavior. This hard-work miracle rewires your brain to a new default pattern.

ROADMAP System® for Performing under Pressure

Recognize your state of mind.

Observe and own any pressure distortions that can initiate a state shift.

Access the ideal state of mind for the task.

Decide which Pressure Management Tool(s) to use.

Map the next best action.

Author that next action.

Program your optimum performance identity.

Recognize your state of mind to effectively enter the mindset of optimum performance for each specific task.

> You create your performance story, including the internal conversation before and during a pressure moment. Each moment, you create what you think, feel, and experience.
>
> With excess pressure and emotional charge, a pause between urge and action creates a

contemplative space in which judgment resides. This place of recognition requires being grounded and centered to become a choice point.

Awareness of emotional triggers and the subsequent state change moves what "just seems to happen" to conscious self-reflective choice.

Recognizing authorship of your state of mind also acknowledges how emotion and behavior are directly connected to your player's performance. Thoughts, feelings, and behaviors are all creations of each moment.

Observe and own your performance story.

Observe and own any pressure distortions that generate anxiety or distraction. By recognizing and owning a pressure moment, you can quickly reset to a centered, grounded state. This step of observing and owning includes labeling of thoughts, feelings, and actions as this moment's creation. Labeling allows you to see the simple straightforward objectivity and ownership of thoughts, feelings, and actions rather than experiencing them as "just happening." This mindfulness practice moves from a passive to an active position internally, with ownership bestowing both acceptance and effectiveness of the created experience.

What remains unconscious will probably be attributed to fate. If you emphasize that you really want something but seem stuck and unable to attain it, ask yourself these questions:

- ☐ What would I observe to know that I really want this?
- ☐ What behavior would demonstrate that I am acting to do that?
- ☐ Is there a component that I can begin right now?
- ☐ How would I feel when I do what I want to do?
- ☐ What is the greater pain if I don't do it?
- ☐ What is the greater pleasure if I do it?

Access and assess the ideal state of mind for the performance task.

> Juxtapose this awareness with assessment of whether your thinking is affected by distortion due to pressure, losing the flow, or moving to an observer position.
>
> Assess the specific performance behaviors and self-talk. Are there limiting beliefs as part of a shadow story? How can you convert them to empowering beliefs?

Decide specifically what to keep, let go, change, and enhance.

> Plan a strategy to use to reboot the performance mindset and zone to optimize performance (see Pressure Management Tools in Chapter 9).

Map the next best action for performance excellence.

> To simply map the next best action, shrink the change to the next step, with the continued question, "Then, what is the next best action?"

Author the ideal response to execute optimum performance.

A strategy needs to be aligned with ideas and purpose. You do not have to be motivated; you only need to have a plan and stick to it. Execute the optimum performance.

- Ideals: core values that motivate and guide
- Purpose: what to accomplish and contribute
- Strategy: the art and science of a plan of action
- Goals: Enter and sustain the specific performance zone.

Program your peak performance identity.

One of the most powerful forces of the human psyche is our persistent return to our core identity, the model of how and who we see ourselves as being. It is necessary to transform this operating model—the bedrock of identity—to correspond with behavioral changes to make change permanent, to transform how you see yourself—doing and being in the performance zone. Incorporating the new behavior as part of a core self—continually assessing evolving skill development and performance results—becomes an ongoing process of self-reflection and recognition. New behavior incorporated into core identity becomes permanent. Change that lasts rewires the brain to a default mode. This automatic sequence becomes a procedural memory to operate automatically as peak performance.

Many approaches to effecting change attempt to do so without considering what change does to a personal narrative, leaving out core identity. As a result, many methods of change are contrary to how the mind and brain work. When you change behavior, a corresponding transformation in your bedrock identity needs to change as well for change to be permanent.

Since much of the performance story operating system is not conscious, its powerful process constructs the story of the performance, of your performance identity, expectations, and ultimately behaviors.

Unlearning and New Performance Habit Learning

Pain brought me to mindfulness, not any desire to reach nirvana or pop out of any chrysalis. It was "unlearning" certain habits and thought patterns hardwired in my brain and walking through my pain, rather than avoiding it, that ultimately put me on a joyful journey of self-discovery.
George Mumford

Ben Fletcher of the University of Hertfordshire, in the United Kingdom, devised a study to get people to break their usual habits. Each day the subjects picked a different option from poles of contrasting behaviors—lively/quiet, introvert/extrovert, reactive/proactive—and behaved according to this assignment. So an introverted person, for example, would act as an extrovert for an entire day. Additionally, twice weekly they had to stretch to behave in a way outside their usual life pattern—eating or reading something they otherwise wouldn't.

The remarkable finding was that after four months, the subjects had lost an average of eleven pounds. Six months later, almost all had kept the weight off. He and his research team were baffled. Their study had nothing to do with dieting or weight loss.

The rationale for the impact of the changes is that requiring people to change routine behavior makes them think about decisions rather than habitually choosing a default mode without consideration. This is story-busting in an indirect way. In having to process decisions actively, they exercised their choice- and decision-making abilities, extending to other choices such as what and what not to eat. Once you become aware that you are actively making choices, you can decide what's in your best interest, what furthers your story, and what doesn't. Fletcher's study became a prototype of choice architecture, to consciously consider creating choices rather than default decisions.

Why is it much easier for a child to learn a foreign language than for an adult? The beginner's mind is the essence of this process of not having to forget or unlearn something to replace it with the newly acquired rather to simply learn something new. For adults, however, much must be unlearned to replace it with the new, like forming a new habit to replace one that already exists. Learning is not the simple acquisition of information but a practiced behavior that replaces beliefs and behaviors already in place. Executing a slightly different forehand in tennis, is not as easy as seeing it instructed and adopting the moves. The old ways of doing things—such as ingrained attachment patterns played out in a business relationship—are already there, well-grooved as an anatomical reality in the brain.

Patterns are developed in the brain by repetitions that create neuronal networks, and every time an action is performed, microscopic rewiring of the brain occurs, making it slightly more grooved each time. After many repetitions, the groove becomes deeper and more automatic.

The more deeply etched the pattern—the deeper the groove—the more challenging it is to change a habit. It takes the same repetition as it did initially, only this time to undo the old pattern and simultaneously etch the new pattern.

A habit engages software created for past experiences. If it is useful, it can tremendously expedite a default and effortless execution. If it is no longer useful and outdated, a new behavior pattern needs to be created. A simple strategy then is to not fight old habits but simply to start new ones. The associations of the past habit become inactive with an immersion in the current, new experience.

This approach also engages a positive focus. When you pick a particular skill, you want to develop such as a tennis backhand stroke, rather than engaging a negative focus, of what is wrong with your current backhand stroke, focus on the ideal stroke you create at this moment. A first step then may be to picture the ideal backhand stroke in full detail, including your experience of it and all the sensory detail that you can. When this visualization in its full experience is revisited over and over, it rewires the brain. Then as you execute the backhand in real time, experience the full feelings in all senses and all somatic register of the backhand to align that with the vision already wired in your brain. You have created a future memory to live into, to actualize with the practice experience. A learning process then shifts from critical judgment from the perspective of an observer of a skill execution to an internal anchoring and execution. Visualizing optimum outcomes combines with being in an optimum performance state to engage the skill behavior. This all occurs at the level of experience, not the level of intellect and conscious judgment. The true transformation occurs when the new experience is incorporated as part of an identity, an alignment with the essence of a performance without observation or judgment. Enjoyment and relaxation into the experience follow.

The Neurochemistry of Unlearning

Unlearning is the process that results in weakening of connections among neurons—a form of reverse neuroplasticity. This unlearning is necessary in our neuronal networks to create room for new connections. The strengthening of some connections while weakening others (unlearning) keep our neural networks from becoming overloaded.

Learning research informs us about optimal approaches to combining learning and unlearning:

- Begin with a question or a story to activate attention and stimulate wanting to know what's next.
- Whatever is new, different, or even surprising captures attention.
- When required to address an uninspiring old topic, change something about it, even if it's the setting or

the application—anything to notify the person's brain of something new and different to grab attention.

- Don't start with a review or summary of what has happened before. Our brains minimize or even ignore information that is old news.

- Frame the new learning as possibility rather than problem, keeping in mind that it is the problem that must be unlearned.

- Engage collaborative discussion and involvement. We learn and recall more when challenged.

- Shrink the change to a next small step for each aspect of new behavior.

- Use multiple modalities in learning to involve more parts of the brain and enhance both learning and memory.

- If reversion to an old habit recurs, interrupt immediately and reestablish the new focus or behavior.

- Remember that an immensely effective means of creating an emotional connection, as well as establishing a memory, is through stories.

- All learning is an emotional process and will become optimized with emotional integration.

Your Mind's Eye: Visualizations and Affirmations

Major James Nesmeth spent seven years as a prisoner of war in North Vietnam. During that time, he was essentially isolated and had no physical activity. Before the war, Nesmeth was an average weekend golfer, breaking 100 by one stroke on two occasions. To preserve his sanity, he learned to visualize golf, which he did every day. He selected his favorite country club. He saw himself dressed in golfing clothes. He experienced everything in great detail. He smelled the fragrance of the trees and the grass and made each stroke with his entire body. After he was released from captivity, he shot a 74 on his first golf outing.

A group of executives asked me to present a seminar on writing a first book. My first question to them was, "How many of you have envisioned your first completed book—exactly what it will look like, the title, how it feels to hold it, seeing it at the bookstore?"

No hands were raised.

My next question: "Have any of you seen a yellow Jeep in the last month?" Of the twenty-four people present, one raised his hand.

I went through a visualization exercise with them:

- Close your eyes and picture a yellow Jeep—the specific detail of how it looks.
- Walk toward it. Walk all around it. Notice the tires, the body, the trim.
- Open the passenger door; feel the cold metal as you grasp the handle.
- Look at the steering wheel, the dash.
- As you sit, notice the secure, firm seat holding your body.
- Smell the interior.
- Look at the dashboard and through the windshield to imagine driving.

- ☐ Start it; hear the motor run; feel the vibration.
- ☐ Grasp the steering wheel and imagine driving.
- ☐ As you turn it off and get out, hear how securely the door closes.
- ☐ As you walk away, look back one more time and take in the entire picture of the yellow Jeep.

I asked them to contact me by e-mail or telephone in the next week if any of them happened to see a yellow Jeep.

In the first three days, twenty-two of the twenty-four executives contacted me to say they had spotted a yellow Jeep. What someone sees—what appears on the radar screen—is determined by belief and assumption. In that particular situation, a yellow Jeep was preprogrammed as possibility. Our possibilities are limited to the ones we allow ourselves to see. They were now seeing both yellow jeeps as well as their first completed book.

The Art of Visualization

Novak Djokovic defeated Roger Federer (7-6, 1-6, 7-6, 4-6, 13-12) to win his second straight Wimbledon men's singles title, his fifth overall. The tennis match lasted just under five hours and ended in the first-ever Wimbledon Gentlemen's Final Tiebreaker. Djokovic, ranked number one in the world, said on the court after receiving his trophy, "This has always been the tournament for me. I used to make the trophies out of different materials in my room as a kid just imagining I would be standing here."

Jack Nicklaus said that 90 percent of a tough shot is the mental picture he creates of how to make it, and 10 percent is the physical swing itself.

Navy SEAL trainer Brandon Webb calls this visualization process "superior mental rehearsal."

A vision crystallizes possibility into a fundamental articulated idea. A vision gives hope possibility—a shape and form—to program your future while rehearsing it. You inhabit the experience of your vision to guide its creation.

A vision serves as inspiration to design ways to realize it. The most successful businesses have a universal vision, one that resonates with each person in the organization. Proven guidelines include the following elements:

- You must construct your own vision.
- The criteria to measure success must be clearly defined.

The combination of physical practice and imagery consistently yields performance superior to physical practice alone.

It is important when using visualization and imagery to avoid negative language or directives, such as what not to do or what to avoid. The unconscious processing part of our midbrain does not know the difference between positive and negative, only focus. The alignment of the energy field of the brain is on the focus, so a focus on "don't turn the ball over" or "don't throw an interception" aligns the energy field with that very issue. Focus on specifically what you want to do. And only that.

Research has repeatedly shown that negative imagery results in performance deterioration. So, direct your imagery and visualization to only positive intention.

The Science of a Vision

Recent positron-emission tomography (PET) scans of the brain have confirmed several things about visualization:

- Visualization brings about actual physical changes in the brain.
- The brain assimilates a mental picture whether the stimulus is actual from the optic nerve or imagined; the brain activates in the same way with a mental image as with an actual image.
- When you repeat a vision of successfully attaining a goal, the act programs neural networks and neuronal pathways to etch the experience more strongly.
- Mental visualization of a complex movement can actually improve performance.

When you program your unconscious, you create a "future memory" to live into. The brain can't tell who conjured it—you or reality. The more detailed your visual image, the more specifically etched your brain will be. We know that by simply picturing a danger, we can trigger the entire body's responses of fight or flight.

You do not make the brain changes permanent unless you incorporate them into your story. Doing so makes it part of who you are—your identity. Otherwise, the change either doesn't register or gets extruded as noise. For example, a phrase that became incorporated as part of an identity was Muhammad Ali's "I am the greatest," introduced in a speech to reporters before his 1964 world title bout with Sonny Liston.

While your unconscious mind cannot tell the difference between something you physically see and something you mentally picture, your conscious mind can. You must incorporate an evolving story to include the successful performance. Otherwise, unconscious messages will delete access to or believability of the imagery.

There are three key elements of effective visualization:

- Specificity about the full experience of achieving the goal: thoughts, feelings, behaviors, sensations.
- Repetition of the success imagery so the neural networks dedicated to that vision become hardwired.
- Conscious incorporation of this new vision into an ongoing story to be ultimately metabolized as part of the self. Otherwise, you will "lose" this vision.

Visualization Exercise

Engage imagery/visualization with a specific goal. This focus on a specific end point and purpose guides intent and personal meaning of the imagery. The visualization/imagery includes the entire scenario of the successful completion scene: visualization, the emotions you will feel, and the conversation that will result.

Envision goals that are Specific, Measurable, Attainable, Relevant, and Time-bound (SMART goals)

- Create positive terms for success.

  Establish your criteria with positive terms that address what you want and what you will do.
- Be specific, simple, concrete.
- Vague and theoretical criteria are not useful, because there is no way to live a theory.

• Be entirely present to your experience of the vision: what you feel, what you think.

- Picture yourself having just succeeded at your goal at a specific time in the future, such as one year from now.
- Create this success experience specific to time, place, and how you would experience yourself and your body through all five senses.
- Hold the energy of the precise outcome you've just achieved, the goals met, and the feelings it brings. Imagine the details of the scene of your success inside and outside, engaging all senses, thoughts, feelings, and bodily experience along with details of the scene. For example, for a successful transaction, include the values and needs fulfilled, the money you have made from it, and the details of what you are doing, such as shaking hands and ushering someone out of your office.
- Carve out a few moments at the beginning and end of each day to “read” this vision.

Affirmations Exercise

Affirmations: The Story to Support Visualizations

According to a recent paper in the Proceedings of the *National Academy of Sciences,* self-affirmations that incorporate what one values and sees as relevant activate the pleasure chemical dopamine to alter the brain’s response to messages, leading to behavior change. Self-affirmations that incorporate core identity of the individual (success, contribution, freedom, etc.) generate significant responsiveness.

Affirmations make visualization a complete story. To achieve a goal, reprogram your automatic pilot with affirmations. Affirmations are positive statements that state the goal as if it has already been achieved. For affirmations to be optimally effective, the following characteristics need to be incorporated.

- Present tense
  Begin with "I am ..." State the goal as if you have already achieved it. "I am skiing every March in Steamboat."
- Positivity
  Your brain will strive to achieve the image you focus on. A positive image is more powerful than ideas
- Personal
  Make your affirmations about your experience and accomplishment. Do not try to change other people's behavior. "I am watching my daughter clean her room" won't work
- Use of all five senses
  Imagine a successful completion with all five senses. For visual, use several lenses, such as wide-angle and close-up; make a complete experience of the successful completion of your goal.
- Emotion
  Include a feeling word ("happily interacting," "peacefully experiencing"). A primary reason we do things is how we imagine we'll feel when we do it.

- Brevity
  Brevity is the soul of wit—and affirmations.
- Specificity
  Clearly focused, specific detail makes it real. No abstractions.
- Action words
  "I am slaloming … driving ... acting ... living ..." If you say "I am going to ..." you will always be on the way.
- Consistency
  As soon as you let up on the disciplined, focused pursuit of a goal, your automatic pilot will revert to the familiar. This is the frustration of not continuing to follow a weight-loss plan and having the weight come back.
- Adding "Or something better"
  "I am enjoying my month spring skiing in Steamboat Springs, or something better." Write each goal and affirmation on a 3x5 card. Read each one at the beginning and the end of each day. Remember to visualize yourself as having already achieved the goal.

How long do you do this?
Until you reach the goal.

How many performance-related goals should you generate affirmations for?
A reasonable number—at least three, maybe more—that you're working on daily.

In this way, you create the complete experience of internal success. You inhabit the experience. An affirmation will initially make you feel uncomfortable, even anxious. With an affirmation that is positive and not yet achieved, you challenge the core belief of your identity and systematically create the template for a new performance story.

Mental Rehearsal

Soviet human rights activist Anatoly Shcharansky spent over nine years imprisoned in the Soviet Union (he was falsely accused of spying for the United States). Shcharansky spent four hundred days of his prison term in a dark, cold isolated "punishment cell" where he played a game of chess in his mind every day. He tracked the board coordinates and positions to generate strategy and develop neural maps to enhance his chess ability. After he was released, he played then-world chess champion Gary Kasparov and beat him.

Mental rehearsal repeatedly imagines a performance in action. When we do this, circuits in the brain reconfigure and, with repetition, rewire to create the imagined act or vision as a physical reality in the brain. With repetition, the neural rewiring configures the thought or vision as the experience. This is a way of truly changing our minds and our brains. In creating a future memory by visualization to change the brain ahead of the experience, neural circuits align with intention and brain reality prior to putting the reality to action. Mental rehearsal installs new neuronal networks and pathways to physiologically pave the way to success scenarios.

Each activation of the experienced new scenario fires and wires new neural circuits more strongly and simultaneously diminishes access to the old story circuits, turns off the old genes, and activates new genes. The visualization, thoughts, and experiences become the new brain engram.

Professionals in any area of performance, including athletic, art, academic, and business, have their own forms and styles of mental rehearsal. Elite performers do more mental practice in the final stages of preparation than their less-successful colleagues.

More than one hundred research studies document the performance benefits of mental practice with imagery.

- Mental rehearsal of each performance sequence creates a neural blueprint of the skill development.
- Mental practice produces the same sequence of activity in the brain as actually performing a task.
- Visualization of a task produces corresponding electrical activity and the small muscle contractions involved in the body's action.
- Mental rehearsal both strengthens and conditions muscle firing and develops neural pathways so that performance behavior becomes more automatic.

Self-Directed Neuroplasticity

Deceptive brain messages can include unfounded fears, worries, rumination, obsession, overthinking, self-blame, reversion to past patterns, or other negative self-talk.

The more you pay attention to the deceptive brain message, the more you etch it into your brain and the more frequent and intense the deceptive brain messages become. The more you engage in the subsequent unwanted behavior, the stronger the brain circuits supporting that behavior become. Just because the deceptive brain message or uncomfortable sensation is present does not mean it has to be acted on.

Four components of self-directed neuroplasticity and choice architecture for making the most informed choices possible in a stepwise fashion can rewire the brain (*You Are Not Your Brain*, Jeffrey Schwartz, MD):

- *Relabel* a deceptive message as an error message from the brain.
- *Reframe* it as a false brain message to not engage it rather than as a directive for action.
- *Refocus* to direct attention away from the deceptive message toward an activity or process that is productive.
- *Revalue* to see the thought, urge, or impulse of the deceptive brain message as an automatic brain activation that can be replaced with a current feeling, thought, or action that is productive.

Each time these four steps are enacted, brain circuits associated with unhealthy habits weaken and desired habits or actions strengthen. These steps emphasize the idea of choice, of how we view events being a product of our own creation. Whatever we think, feel, and experience, we create each moment.

Summary Principles of Changing Mind, Brain, and Behavior to Enhance Player Performance

- ☐ Begin with what the person already knows.
- ☐ Highlight positive attributes—existing neuronal networks (natural talents, behaviors, and patterns) to encourage their practice.
- ☐ Don't focus on mistakes. Focus will enhance neuronal etching, so it should be on useful habits.
- ☐ Correct mistaken couplings. Understand and build on existing networks.
- ☐ Let sleeping dogs and old unuseful networks lie. Don't focus on understanding why.
- ☐ Help the person create self-talk scripts to navigate.
- ☐ Help the player recognize and own experiences.
- ☐ Determine what to keep, let go, enhance, and avoid.
- ☐ Repetition changes your mind and your brain.
- ☐ The brain has an intrinsic desire to create novel connections.
- ☐ Give attention to a new experience or a new way of doing things consistently and repetitively.

SECTION III. PERFORMANCE OPTIMIZATION

Basketball coach Mike Krzyzewski spoke about his concern for his star players. "When I am coaching my Duke team, I need to be the best player's best friend. Being the best player is a lonely position. Even though you get accolades, no matter how good a team you have, there is always some level of jealousy. Always." Often exceptional achievement results in those star performers being left alone and coaches focusing on the low performers, taking for granted the continued excellence of the high achievers. According to Krzyzewski, that is a mistake. "Leadership is not just to let the star produce but to be a friend of the star, to motivate the star. Your team is going to go a lot further if your stars push ahead and everybody else must work to catch up."

The neuroscience of performance is based on a bedrock foundation of understanding both mind and brain. The anatomy of arousal involves a balance of neurochemicals that constitute the "DNA" of peak performance: Dopamine, the pleasure neurotransmitter, Norepinephrine, the neurochemical regulating attention and alertness, and Acetylcholine, the neurochemical most involved in the actual peak performance itself, released at a crucial time of new learning and brain neuroplasticity for focus and activation of optimum learning machinery.

Performance problems often have more to do with mindset than with motivation, intelligence, or skill. For a performer in any endeavor (athlete, surgeon, executive) who has practiced essentially the same thousands of hours as the next person, optimum outcome is determined more by sustaining a specific performance mindset. Performance under pressure requires pressure management tools and systematic strategies. The most common success completion issues of choking, sandbagging, self-handicapping, and burnout are detailed, along with their remedies.

“Playing to win” demands a different mindset than “playing not to lose.” You’ll see a detailed strategy for “playing to win,” including 34 different ways to distinguish performance experts from amateurs.

Extreme success breeds specific challenges: performance plateaus, invincibility syndrome, loss of perspective and objectivity, distraction and self-indulgence, summit syndrome, and success intoxication. These success traps can test one’s mettle as surely as the strongest adversary. Staying at the top is both art and neuroscience.

Chapter 8. Optimum Performance Strategies

Knowledge is only a rumor until it lives in the muscle.
The Asaro Tribe of Papua New Guinea

Self-Talk and Performance

A CEO I'll call Dan experienced a tragedy at his company in the form of a serious accident that resulted in on-the-job injuries and a death. In the three months after the accident, he had stress-related symptoms of losing sleep, depleted energy, and preoccupation with safety. He recognized that his responses hampered his effectiveness as an executive and his ability to provide the leadership that his company needed, and he contacted me for executive mentor coaching.

Eventually I asked Dan what went through his mind the moment he woke up. His immediate answer: "What could go wrong today?" He wondered what he could do to ensure safety for his company, how he could stop feeling helpless, how he could assure the group that there would be no more accidents, how he could mitigate any potential future danger.

I explained that we are always asking ourselves questions, whether we are conscious of them, from the moment we wake up. And this internal conversation sets in motion a mindset to initiate the day, to build on. This inner dialogue at stressful times can include questions like “What’s going to happen today?” “Will I be able to handle it?” and “What am I most afraid of?”

He recognized that the negative mindset that began his day for the three months since the event had been essentially the same and had set the tone for both himself and his corporation. Not only his executive team but each employee had embraced his concern. He knew he had to do something but wasn’t quite sure what to do, as nothing seemed to work for very long.

I suggested that sometime during the day or evening before he went to bed, he writes down three questions that would put him in an empowered, positive state of mind, questions that would focus on his effectiveness and instantly boot up a state of mind of confidence and mastery. And to answer those questions each morning as soon as he woke up.

The next week at our session, he immediately reported the difference those questions had made. By shifting consciously to positive self-talk, he booted up a positive mindset that built on itself throughout the day.

This initial reframing of his self-narrative to direct the power of focus to launching a positive state of mind became a model that he had passed on, directly and indirectly, to his organization. He noticed, within days, the impact it had on his executive team and how this change trickled down through the organization.

How can self-talk enhance performance?

Researcher Daniel Wegner found that stress usually causes a reversion to avoid the negative—a "Do not …" internal instruction. Since the unconscious brain is only aware of focus and not positive or negative valuation, this unfortunately brings about whatever the "Do not ..." focuses on.

Specific self-talk needs to be matched to the endeavor. Before a keynote, “relaxed and powerful” may engage an optimum mindset, whereas the distance runner may choose “steady pace.” What we say to ourselves during challenging moments can have an impact on how we perform. Self-talk can be one of two types: motivational or instructional. Motivational self-talk can function to increase effort: “I am going all out,” or to enhance confidence: “I got this.”

Dr. Samuel Marcora and his colleagues demonstrated the effectiveness of a brief self-talk intervention. Volunteers completed a cycling test to exhaustion. Then, before another cycling test two weeks later, half of them were given guidance on positive self-talk while the other half were not. The self-talk phrases included “feeling good” and, later in the race, “push through this.” The emphasis for the self-talk group was to have the phrase fit their style and construction. In this second cycling test, the self-talk group persisted 18 percent longer than the controlled group. This showed how a simple self-talk can influence experience and the resulting performance. Many other studies involving more numbers and more sophistication have proved the validity of this concept.

A sizable body of research has shown the value of engaging in self-talk, specifically to objectively frame a situation. Professional athletes need to get grounded and centered after every play, particularly after an emotionally stimulating play. We are just beginning to study and understand the functions of inner speech, of talking to ourselves silently in our heads. Self-talk can anticipate, self-regulate, and motivate. A brief cue word or gesture can instantly reset us to an ideal performance state.

We always engage in self-talk, always ask questions, whether we are consciously aware of this process. The first step is to be aware of the running commentary of self-talk. This recognition and awareness reframe to focus on self-directing positive, enhancing questions for a success mindset.

Positive self-talk can help to enter an optimum mindset for a specific task to sustain focus for flow and cognitive rhythm.

Self-Talk: First and Third Person

A study of Olympic gold medalists found two traits that set superachievers apart: complete confidence and self-talk for entering the state of mind of confidence. Elite performers rigorously monitor their self-talk as well as their states of mind. Examples of audible self-talk by athletes include Serena Williams's shouting, "Come on, Serena," and LeBron James's speaking to himself out loud.

First- and third-person self-talk can be effective, with first person being the initiator of action, the internal point of self-reference, and third person serving as the observer, an observing mentor or observing ego to reflect and self-correct.

Brain imaging shows that first- and third-person images and narratives stimulate the brain. Both imagining and watching yourself doing something stimulates the brain in the exact way that experiencing it does. This can amount to an effective component of practice. Imagining doing something rather than just intending to do it activates the brain and makes follow-through more likely. The more specifically you imagine something, the more likely you are to do it.

A subtle variation of self-talk can serve the defensive purpose of distancing or disavowing an aspect of experience. When you speak of your experience, you usually use first person, saying "I" or "we." When you notice yourself moving to second person and beginning with "You," that is usually the instant there is some discomfort that you want to distance yourself from or disavow, as if disconnecting from your core self. Notice in interviews by the press that when someone is uncomfortable with a situation, they shift to refer to themselves in the second person. Whenever this occurs with a client in coaching, immediately engage a reflection of the experience and what it means to more effectively deal with it rather than distancing it.

At times, talking to yourself in the third person can transcend the emotion of the moment or even an emotional state. An example is the highly charged career decision that LeBron James made about leaving Cleveland to go to Miami to pursue championships. As he struggled with whether to leave his hometown Cavaliers and join the Miami Heat to move himself to a new level in his career, he described his thought process. "One thing I didn't want to do was make an emotional decision. I wanted to do what's best for LeBron James and to do what makes LeBron James happy." He initially referred to himself in the first person, but when he discussed how he wanted to avoid an emotional decision, he switched to the third person, "LeBron James."

Research shows that using the third person this way is an effective technique for distancing yourself from stress, anxiety, frustration, or sadness to regulate emotional state and enhance objectivity. It can also reframe stressful situations as challenges and opportunities rather than as threats.

Self-Talk to Enhance Commitment

In the six-month Navy SEAL training, more than two-thirds of the candidates will drop out in the first eight weeks. Pain, sleep deprivation, and frequent harsh wet and cold conditions effectively ensure that, on average, only 25 percent of the candidates will eventually make it through. What determines who makes it? Instructors observe that there is one true predictor of which candidates will ultimately succeed: *wanting it the most*. Commitment. Candidates who make a full commitment to their goal of becoming a Navy SEAL differ in that they decide ahead of time that quitting is not an option regardless of the challenges. This commitment increases their chances more than strength, agility, speed, and intelligence.

Of all factors that lead to it, commitment is ultimately and finally a behavior. Commitment is an "I will." Commitment is not the same as motivation. Commitment guides intentional direction and purposeful practice. A commitment of goal completion "no matter what," regardless of how you feel, is necessary for success. Otherwise, there can be any number of reasons sufficient to justify scaling back or rationalizing stopping early.

There will always come a time when there will be a choice between emotions driving behavior and commitment to a plan driving behavior. How you direct emotion can make a huge difference in fulfilling a commitment. A commitment to persevere is, particularly for the most difficult moments, not the easier or more convenient one. This is what separates elite performance from everything else. As Dr. Eddie O'Connor said in consulting with a hockey team at halftime after a challenging first half with numerous personal fouls, "You can get mad and fight or you can get mad and play hockey. You can't do both."

Commitment is a choice you make each moment each day.

In another application, a study showed that sales agents who score in the top 10 percent for optimism were able to sell 88 percent more than the most pessimistic bottom 10 percent. This is not about skill or ability but about perseverance based on the story of an internal conversation.

The most resilient individuals are those who create a self-talk about failure's being an anomaly, and they keep going. Martin Seligman at the University of Pennsylvania found that what measured as helplessness was really the pessimism of the self-talk that "I'm not cut out for this" or "I'm not really good at these things." This helplessness can be converted with proper framing and self-talk into optimism. Research validates that optimism is associated with better health, a longer life, improved survival of cardiovascular disease, and more positive opportunities to result in happiness.

Seligman found that pessimists' stories and optimists' stories diverge in this way: Pessimists believe that bad events will last a long time, are universal, and are basically their own fault. Optimists believe that bad events are temporary and look for a specific cause and remedy rather than blaming themselves.

Our self-talk stories keep us going or stop us. Our stories need to be greater than our pessimism or our pain. And especially greater than a story line that has become part of a behavior and attachment pattern of not being able to do it.

Self-awareness becomes a crucial component of both monitoring and understanding this process. Self-awareness determines whether we can objectively question and understand our behavior, as well as take in different perspectives, including those of coaches.

The most common reason you can't have what you want is the story you tell yourself about why you can't have it.

Framing Self-Talk for Resilience

Angela Duckworth's research at the University of Pennsylvania shows that those with grit—the fortitude to stick with tasks—relies in large part on the self-talk of the story to give it meaning. It is estimated that we say between three hundred and a thousand words to ourselves every minute. When we speak to ourselves positively ("I can do it") rather than negatively ("I can't do this anymore"), it has a major impact on resilience—the mental toughness to keep going.

Inner dialogues can facilitate rebound from failure. Engineering Professors David Franklin and Daniel

Wolpert have identified five mechanisms of brain operation that go into action when someone successfully bounces back from failure or circumvents it. Each mechanism has a specific corresponding brain function to allow us to directly access an inner dialogue to rebound from failure with resilience and transform to success.

1. Redirection of negative feedback
   Whether external or internal, it focuses energy in the brain in a negative way.
   Self-reflection questions: What can I learn from this? What are the possibilities here (rather than the problems)?

2. Creation of obstacles
   Consider that the obstacle you are experiencing is not something external to simply strategize a way to avoid or overcome, but that the obstacle is not there until you create it through the way you see or frame something. To say this a different way, an obstacle is the unconscious mnemonic of desire. Show me an obstacle and I'll show you a desire. When you are ready to consider that you are creating the obstacle, you are ready to consider the possibility of not creating it.
   Self-reflection question: What would it be like to not create the obstacle and instead put the energy into what I want?

3. Use of systematic forecasting
   We each use invisible brain algorithm to predict the future. Our brain creates new pathways and networks for anything we repeat, and this default mode saves energy. These hard-wired patterns become predictive because they create the story that

we anticipate. To preempt this automatic system, we have to consciously self-reflect to see if the software that was developed at an earlier time even for a similar context is applicable to the current situation. Or if it's outdated and needs revision.
Self-reflection question: Is my usual pattern optimum for this current situation?

4. Assessment of the current model
Self-reflect to assess the effectiveness of what you're doing and if it is working. This requires, at times, disruption of automatic expectations rather than continuing to inhabit the story that we want to believe.
Self-reflection question: Is this plan really working?

5. Direction to an output channel.
No matter how much we acquire information, study, and learn, it is by putting it into action—using the output channel—that we not only enhance effectiveness but create a performance story.
Self-reflection question: What do I next need to put into action?

Self-Talk Exercise
Empowering and Limiting Words

Words can change your brain and your body. Our bodies listen to the words used at a subtle level. Words are powerful in that they set both expectations and limitations about how much we're capable of.

Seligman has found that optimistic expectations become a significant component of actual performance.

Beliefs directly affect the outcome of efforts and performance results.

Create a list of empowering words.

Words and language are a part of mental software that drive behavior. A simple example of building an "out" such as to say, "I'll try…" can be reframed in a more powerful way as a commitment: "I will." Exceptional performers become aware of limiting beliefs, as beliefs can frame a mindset.

Examples of empowering words:

- *Powerful*
- *Accomplished*
- *Unstoppable*

We set intentions by using empowering or limiting words—and our unconscious follows. The unconscious does not know the difference between negative and positive, just the focus. This form of unconscious programming can have powerful effects either negatively or positively.

Create a list of limiting words.

Whenever you hear yourself thinking or saying any limiting word, immediately delete and reframe to an empowering word and thought. This form of immediate biohacking can be extremely effective in cuing your radar to be aware of a default mode.

Examples of limiting words that can boot up limiting performance:

- *Try*
- *Can't*

• *Bad*

Our unconscious listens to the label, not to negative or positive.

Peak Experience and Peak Performance

If you are about to give a presentation to an audience of several hundred peers, what do you consider your best immediate preparation: to calm yourself or to feel excited?

Alison Wood Brooks, professor at Harvard Business School, asked several hundred people this question. Ninety-one percent thought the best preparation was to calm themselves.

Dr. Brooks then created an experiment to examine this question. She asked half the group to calm themselves before a presentation to a large group of people and the other half to embrace their anxiety and excitement. Those who told themselves "I am excited" handled the pressure better and were more confident and effective in their presentations. Independent raters determined that the group of more excited presenters showed greater confidence, competence, and persuasiveness than those who simply tried to calm down. The mindset framing anxiety as excitement helped them perform better under pressure.

A significant number of studies find that common psychological characteristics of an optimum performance state include:

- Confidence
- Full concentration

- Focus on the present task
- Positive expectations about performance
- Strong determination and commitment
- Feeling energized and relaxed
- Expecting success
- Feeling a sense of mastery and effectiveness
- Mobilized and organized energy

Peak experiences are personal moments of lasting positive affect, an exciting and fulfilling high point of an experience that is unusually intense and meaningful.

A flashbulb moment of peak experience serves as exemplary moments to positively highlight and represent an entire set of experiences. These instances can serve as organizer and motivator for other performance-based activities.

Peak experiences, like peak performances, are most likely to occur in a state of flow, the sustained state of mind that allows access to the execution of a skill developed by deliberate practice.

Mastering all aspects of pressure situations can include awareness of thoughts, feelings, and emotional triggers that could disrupt focus and state.

Disruptions in optimal performance most often correlate with loss of concentration in the moment, loss of focus on the task, distraction by some specific interference, and self-doubt. Excessive focus on a competitor or team outcome or score can impede performance, as can over-arousal and under-arousal. Focused attention is a premier psychological skill for performance. A lack of focus, even temporarily, can devastate performance and even risk injury. Compromise occurs when a performer's attention shifts from immersion in the flow of the skilled performance in any way.

Optimum performance requires regulating and sustaining focused attention. Attention includes concentration on a specific target and focus on the actions determined by the performer. Attention has multiple dimensions, including alertness, accessing a state for optimum performance, then a specific and selective engagement on the flow state while ignoring all other information.

The Quiet Eye

Your mind is like a camera that focuses on one among an almost infinite number of possibilities. The Quiet Eye is simply close-up attention to the final step in a performance sequence. Specific focus on this one aspect quiets the entire system for optimal execution of a task.

Eye-tracking research on the "quiet eye" shows that for a precise motor task like free-throw shooting, putting, or tying a surgical knot, experts maintain quiet eye 62 percent longer than nonexperts. Quiet eye focus specifically increases precision. Dr. Joan Vickers, professor of kinesiology at the University of Calgary, showed a free-throw accuracy increase of 22 percent after training. She emphasized focusing on a single spot on the hoop, such as midway between the front and center, and continuing to do so through the shot. Begin at least a full second before initiating the shot and don't shift eye focus for even a nanosecond. A quick fluid motion without losing focus on the quiet eye spot becomes most successful.

Academic and business performers can learn a great deal about applying the quiet eye concept from research in athletic settings. Focus aligns the energy field of the brain and has the functional role of readying the entire system for the next step, especially important when performing under pressure.

Quiet eye training enhances the default motor system execution of skills for a specific target. Sports science shows the benefits of choosing the best visual target for purposeful and goal-directed eye movements. For example, when basketball players miss free shots, it's often because they briefly move focus from the spot on the rim where the ball is going to the ball itself. Also, it's been found that when soccer players miss a penalty shot, it may be because they briefly shifted their focus from the ball's targeted destination just inside the goalpost to the goalkeeper, which obscures the target. In a similar way, an executive can be sidetracked by an emotional reaction to a colleague.

The more important the task, the more important the quiet eye becomes. Practice under pressure enhances performance under pressure. Studies show that high-stress practice for everyone from basketball players to police officers far outpaces low-anxiety training to establish and maintain an output channel of performance and quiet eye focus.

Routine and Specific Ritual for Enhancing Performance

Can a specific ritual enhance performance?

In several studies, athletes who used a pre-performance routine performed better than those who did not.

- A pre-performance routine can boot up the specific mindset for the skill to be performed. An example is the mantra for a free throw.
- Warm-up routines enable preparation and access to a state of mind of optimum performance, whether for a specific athletic endeavor, a keynote presentation, or an executive board meeting.
- During a performance, default routines need to be automatic to sustain immersion in flow.
- Post-performance routines promote not only recovery but reflection and review of the performance for the sake of ongoing improvement.

Effective focus for optimum performance includes some fundamental elements:

- A decision to focus on only the performance itself.
- Concentration on thinking and doing the same specific thing.
- Attending to only those aspects that are under your control.
- An outward focus to counter performance anxiety, preoccupation, or distracting thoughts.

- Avoidance of internal focus, which can introduce doubt, worry, self-criticism, and hypervigilance.

A ritual may include one component of the mantra of neural conditioning, such as a word or phrase, to immediately access an optimum state of mind.

Superstitious behavior rituals are designed to bind anxiety and may not work well as a performance routine. A superstitious ritual may work temporarily but can distract by investing attention in an irrelevant object or action, as if it is a causal link with performance. A superstitious ritual can decrease anxiety and enhance confidence temporarily. However, it may not be the best or most direct way to enhance performance. A performance routine can be a specific and beneficial ritual and can be distinguished from superstitious actions that are repetitive yet distinct from technical performance. The primary difference is that a superstitious act emerges from a desire to influence or control the uncontrollable, especially in the face of uncertainty. Superstition is a form of magical thinking that can be a pre-performance routine but needs to be assessed for improvement vs. anxiety-binding.

The key to optimum performance is to enter an optimum state of mind for the specific performance, a state that contains the software and hardwiring of the execution of that specific skill. A routine or ritual can guide for performance execution.

Evidence-Based Tactics for Building Resilience in Performance

More than education, more than experience, more than training, a person's level of resilience will determine who succeeds and who fails. That is true in the cancer ward, it is true in the Olympics, and it is true in the boardroom.
Dean M. Becker

General Manager Theo Epstein guided the Boston Red Sox to their first World Series victory in eighty-six years. Then he agreed in 2011 to take the reins as president of operations for the Chicago Cubs, whose last World Series championship was in 1908. The Cubs then won in 2016, 108 years later. Widely touted as having an innate and rare intelligence for deconstructing a situation to its simplest form and generating strategic possibilities, he was asked how he decides what he looks for in putting together a team. He indicated that he scouts the person more than the player. He said the first thing he wants to know about any potential player is how he has handled adversity.

Why are some people able to maintain high self-esteem and self-sufficiency despite adversities that lead others to give up and lose hope?

Resilience grows from converting mistakes into lessons. By reflecting on and learning from mistakes, we convert a regrettable experience into a learning experience. Resilience is a biological- and psychological-based ability to regulate emotional states, especially during stress. Success in any arena hinges on resilience. Management of setbacks to productively progress becomes an essential process of optimal performance. A resilient individual is not someone who avoids stress but someone who learns how to effectively master it and optimize performance while doing so. Any endeavor, especially those of significance, will involve both setbacks and stress. The developed resilience of reacting to setbacks and stress often determines the magnitude of success.

The ability to regulate states of mind and manage emotions is central to establishing resilience. Two approaches shown in recent research to regulate states of mind and enhance resilience are cognitive reappraisal and mindfulness meditation.

Cognitive reappraisal reframes from a negative to a positive, from problem to possibility to reinterpret the meaning of an adverse event to see it as a challenge and an opportunity. A Mount Sinai School of Medicine study of Vietnam prisoners of war found that those who had actively reappraised their imprisonment to find meaningful ways in which to grow stronger and more resilient showed the most adaptive responses.

What is the role of tenacity?

It's not that I am so smart, it's that I stick with problems longer.
Einstein

Tenacity involves establishing meaningful goals and strategies for achieving them. Motivation is enhanced by specific goals. Focus and concentration are enhanced by creating specific strategies to reach them. Stepwise strategies include setting initiatives for each goal and the next best action for each initiative.

Some characteristics of those with tenacity:

- Staying power
- Discipline
- Ability to overcome challenges
- Mental acuity to reason and conceptualize problems
- Innovation to invent new ways of proceeding
- Sense of teamwork
- Self-confidence to proceed relentlessly

Stepwise goals enhance focus as well as create a sustained situation of new experiences of effectiveness.

What are the primary factors of sustaining and intensifying effort in performance?

Effort intensity is dependent on one primary aspect more than all others: perceived progress. Business school researchers in Singapore and the United States studied more than one hundred early-stage entrepreneurs to determine progress made toward ultimate goals and perceptions of their effort intensity. The business school entrepreneurs who believed they were making steady progress worked harder. Then the primary thing that facilitated that sense of making progress was studied: setting smaller, attainable goals. The perception of progress was a stepwise incremental experience of sustained effectiveness.

When you create a map, you know where you are, where you're going, how to measure progress along the way, and what's detour and distraction. The steps are an incremental system to the reference point of goals. Effectiveness occurs with each small incremental step. Achievable goals enhance the energy to pursue them.

Rather than a focus on a big-picture objective, this is the system that works when change is needed.

How do you train for mental toughness?

The question isn't who's going to let me; it's who is going to stop me.
Ayn Rand

Mental toughness refers to the psychological edge that enables more determined, confident, and better performance under pressure. Determination and focus constitute its foundation, and it incorporates the commitment to both practice and perform "no matter what."

Mental toughness includes consistently bringing focus back to the performance after inevitable distractions or missteps. Much like the principle of mindful meditation to focus on breathing and accepting that your mind will inevitably wander, the most important thing is to bring the focus back to breathing.

Mental toughness can be developed and improved to create an edge in any kind of performance. Consistency is the key to reengaging focus again and again.

Mastery of performance pressure means effectively managing your thoughts and feelings, performing with intention, and sustaining focus despite temptations to give in to distractions or emotional reactions.

Dr. Rob Harmison, in a meta-analysis of research on mental toughness, found these components to be essential: confidence, intrinsic motivation, effective dealing with adversity/failure, overcoming emotional and physical pain, and successfully managing anxiety and pressure. Managing tremendous success with a balance of focus and perspective is its own challenge and will be addressed in the final chapter.

Resilience training consists of building mental toughness to focus on achievement while creating a systematic way to avoid thinking traps such as letting a single setback or failure become defining. Building signature strengths occurs by reflecting on what you learn about yourself and identifying the strengths developed through your practice. Specifically, developing those strengths contributes to successful completion of a goal.

Enhancing mental toughness is achieved by focusing and developing strengths as well as fostering strong relationships that provide a supportive framework for competency and success.

Brain training for less tangible factors like mental fatigue can contribute to optimum performance. Research shows that when we train the brain to become accustomed to mental fatigue, it can adapt to sustain an optimal performance and develop its own kind of resilience, much as the body can. This involves a seemingly radical training of improving endurance performance by systematically focusing on mental tasks such as repeated computer exercises. Simply put, physical training works both for the body and the mind, for both physical and mental endurance. Brain endurance training needs to parallel physical endurance training.

Mental Energy Restoration for Optimal Performance

Almost everything will work again if you unplug it for a few minutes.
Anne Lamott

How is periodic rest a part of deliberate practice?

When Athenian culture was flourishing in ancient Greece, Plato and his contemporaries didn't separate physical from intellectual education and development. These wise philosophers were on to something that we are now rediscovering. Sound mind and sound body go hand in hand.

At times we may view rest as passive, such as when an athlete sees it as "not training." Called “unfocus” by Dr. Srini Pillay, this activity recognizes rest and unfocused time as something that supports achievement to create a framework that is both effective and proactive. In this reframe, rest becomes a crucial component of a workout or work itself. This kind of rest is an active process both psychologically and physically. Since we make our best efforts in intense periods of sustained focus and work, followed by short breaks, the breaks become a part of the process.

In a study measuring specific tasks of sustained creativity, those who took a six-minute walk outdoors increased their creative output after the walk by 60 percent (Gilford's Alternate Use Test). Those who took a six-minute walk indoors increased their productivity by 40 percent. Walking disengages focused concentration, allowing tapping into unconscious processes, including creativity. The Top Down System rests, and the Bottom Up System takes over.

Recently it has been shown that taking a two-minute walk every hour addresses physical health in particular ways. One study showed that short walks done consistently reduced the risk of premature death by 33 percent.

Peak experiences require periodic timeouts, interludes of unfocus to reboot and refresh. The energy of performance, whether intellectual or physical, can best be achieved with full immersion and intensity for a period of time and can be sustained for optimum results with periodic planned segments of restoration. A relaxation response break creates a structure for the necessary downtime, the unfocused restoration of energy and crispness.

These periodic planned moments of internal rest lead to enhanced immersion and output. This time may be filled with self-reflection and self-awareness and create a tool for engaging and monitoring optimum performance.

Ericksson found that great performers usually work in chunks of sixty to ninety minutes and then take a break. In various industries and types of work, chunks of work followed by short breaks consistently promote effective and sustained results.

Findings of best work-rest ratios include:

- The Draugiem Group found that their workers in intellectual endeavors did best with a fifty-two-minute work time and a seventeen-minute break.

- Workers in a meat processing plant most efficiently worked fifty-one minutes on and nine minutes off each hour.
- Agricultural workers were most productive in seventy-five-minute cycles of one hour on and fifteen minutes off.
- Other studies looking at highly cognitive work found that fifty-one minutes of work and seven minutes off generated the best work outcome.

Play—also related to the process of unfocus—engages the prefrontal cortex to nurture cognitive functions, improving reasoning ability. Einstein emphasized that his ability to generate profound insights into the nature of the universe was a result of his engagement with play. For him, this was a period of unfocus in which he disengaged with the intense intellectual work to balance a combination of work and play.

Failing Well

Smith College's Wurtele Center for Work and Life initiated a directive to de-stigmatize failure and foster student resilience. When students enroll in Rachael Simmons's program "Failing Well," they receive a certificate of failure when they begin. It reads, "You are hereby authorized to screw up, bomb, or fail at one or more relationships, hookups, friendships, texts, exams, extracurriculars, or any other choices associated with college… and still be a totally worthy, utterly excellent human being."

This permission slip to fail puts the impossibility of perfection into focus. "Perfect," "more," and other intangibles are not goals, as they are impossible to attain.

They simply masquerade as a goal but ultimately lead to disappointment.

This is only one of several initiatives designed to foster resilience and to counter a fear of taking risks. Faculty at Harvard and Stanford earlier created the term *failure-deprived* to describe students who were struggling to cope with even temporary setbacks in their expectations.

Chapter 9. Sustaining Peak Performance under Pressure

Self-Regulation and Optimum Performance

During the 2013 NBA playoffs, LeBron James sat courtside, eyes closed. Despite the energy and chaos swirling around him, he turned his focus inward and kept it there until he returned to the game.

We now know that performance gaps have more to do with mindset than they do with motivation, intelligence, or skill. When a performer in any endeavor (athlete, surgeon, executive etc.) has put in the same tens of thousands of hours as the next person, different outcomes trace their origins to different states of mind. Thus, once a certain level of competence has been achieved, the most important "success variable" becomes the ability to master one's state of mind to sustain performance flow.

If there is any realm of human endeavor where state of mind is constantly challenged, it's sports. Players must create a sort of mental space between never-ending stimuli—personal fouls, physical assaults, trash-talk and rule-breaking—and the natural instinct to react instantaneously, instead of remaining "in the zone" and going on with the performance.

Focused attention must remain consistent throughout the performance. Distractions that would throw an average player off his or her game—personal fouls, physical assaults, name-calling—must be ignored.

Internal distractions like self-doubt must be dealt with in the same way.

States of mind, including the ones we call "moods," contain unconscious biases. When we feel happy or enthusiastic, for example, we tend to take more risks (including financial risks). Sadness makes us lean toward safer bets. Disappointment and sadness tend to make us focus on negative information and analytic rather than creative or intuitive thinking.

Regulate States of Mind

Each state of mind is like a specific software program containing a set of particular emotions, memories, mental models and behavioral patterns. Our minds constantly monitor and interpret the world around us, to give us a running account of what's happening, what it means, and what to do about it. Mindsets include the powerful beliefs we use to create stories about ourselves.

A key element of mastery in any field is the ability to determine the best state of mind for that activity—and to create and sustain that state of mind in the face of various physical and emotional triggers and charged situations.

For any given situation, there are three components of experience and response:

- State
- Story
- Strategy

State management is the most important aspect of both practice and performance: choosing the mindset that matches the desired outcome.

Story is how you organize what you do; the theme and storyline of your quest to reach a goal. For Martin Luther King, his story was, “I have a dream.”

Strategy is the specific plan to execute a successful performance. Strategy is not a beginning but a process that includes constant re-evaluation and course correction along the way.

Mindset Mastery

The way you view something changes your body’s response to it. Elite performers channel heightened attention to energize optimum performance.

Individuals and teams (business, sports, etc.) like to think they do their best when the stakes are highest and the future rests on the immediate outcome of whatever it is they’re doing. But the reality is somewhat different. Harvard Professor Heidi Gardner’s extensive study of teams revealed several repeating patterns:

- Teams that become caught up in the risks of failure rather than the pursuit of excellence may revert to standard and safe practices, instead of seeking original solutions.
- When teams face significant performance pressure, they tend to rely on high-status members rather than expert members.
- Excess pressure often causes strongly favored competitors to squander big leads and/or lose the competition.

Vast amounts of research on performance have consistently shown that most people perform below their capacity when under pressure, which erodes behavioral skills unless managed in a systematic way. This is true for everything from parallel parking to Olympic competition. Unless pressure is strategically regulated:

- Attention, judgment, and decision-making are adversely affected.
- Performance incentives and motivational enhancement can camouflage pressure.
- Teams become increasingly focused on problems rather than the pursuit of excellence.

Stress is any situation with too many demands and too few resources—energy, time, or money—to meet them.

Pressure is any situation where something of importance is at stake and relies upon the outcome of a performance.

While the learning zone and the performance zone are distinct, the training and performance states of mind are the same. You may have pulled a caffeinated all-nighter in preparation for a college exam, only to find your brain unable to access some of that information because your exam state of mind was not the same as your study state of mind. Like that rat in the maze.

Success most often has to do with how someone manages an internal state under pressure-inducing circumstances. Those who manage well, perform better. Those who don't, tend to become more physiologically activated, mentally rigid, and impulsive.

While we can't eliminate pressure in every situation, there are pressure management techniques we can use to minimize its effects. After surveying 30,000 people across thirty different countries, researcher Robert Epstein found that the single most effective approach to pressure management is to have a specific plan that makes each step along the journey simple, specific, and tangible.

Is there a mindset to improve performance under stress?

When Olympic gold medal rower Greg Searle was asked whether success was worth the sacrifice, he said. "I never made any sacrifices. I made choices."

The way we think about anything has a profound effect on the way we perceive it, and what we do about it. Our mindset towards stress determines whether we will engage it, and then how we specifically respond, emotionally and physically.

Performing Under Pressure

Anyone can hold the helm when the sea is calm.
Publilius Syrus

Nathan was a well-known nonfiction writer with a book on the New York Times bestseller list. Even so, he found himself experiencing writer's block. By the time he called me, he hadn't written a word for eight weeks. I asked him to walk me through his writing process, step by step. I also asked to hear his internal dialogue. He said that when he sat down to write, "I get anxious and begin doing a lot of different things other than writing. Then I start wondering if I can produce another bestseller or was it just a one-time happening."

After exploring the details of his process distractions, I observed, "It sounds like you get really excited—maybe more so than ever—about immersing yourself in the passion you've always wanted to experience." When Nathan confirmed this, I continued. "When you read the excitement as anxiety, it puts you in your old story where anxiety equals danger. In that story, distracting yourself was a way of regulating the tension."

Nathan's experience of anxiety coupled with his coping by distraction were part of his old story. When he accurately recognized his current experience as excitement, he could sustain his creative state. He also reframed his excitement as validation of this process and as a signpost of progress –and wrote an even bigger bestseller.

Performance Anxiety

Bill Russell vomited before every NBA game yet won eleven championships. He regularly reframed his nausea as part of his preparation ritual—a steppingstone to playing great basketball.

Everyone—even seasoned pros—experience "nerves" and the physical symptoms that come with them: rapid heartbeat, trembling sweaty hands, a sinking feeling in the gut, sometimes even difficulty breathing.

Recasting stress as a challenge can have advantages.

One study found that elite performers viewed stress as a challenge and a measure of their commitment to optimize performance—while less successful athletes viewed stress as something to get around, overcome, or simply tolerate while moving on. Response to stress as opportunity and challenge can lead to better performance.

Trying to prevent, avoid or ignore stress "frames" it as a sign that something's wrong. And it takes emotional and physical energy to fight off the feeling of anxiety that comes with that—energy that could be better spent on the task at hand. Simply telling yourself, "I am excited," shifts your mind from seeing stress as a threat to overcome (anxiety, fear)—to seeing it as something to engage. Instead of trying to chase it away, elite performers welcome and channel stress to drive their performance to ever-higher levels.

Part of this involves disengaging from stakes. If an athlete or other performer is thinking about money or fame, they're not focusing on the performance. The part of the brain responsible for peak performance knows nothing of these things, so any focus on them is mere distraction. Regardless of stakes, the peak performer must become fully immersed in the performance itself.

Focusing only on the next step of the performance turns off the conscious brain, disengages observation and judgment, and allows us to enter (and remain in) the performance zone.

Any disruption of "flow state" by negative self-talk, fear of mistakes, or looking too many steps ahead alters the mental state necessary for continued high-level performance. The mind must remain focused and be able to regain that focus if momentarily distracted. Everyone is different, so this process may vary somewhat from person to person. What doesn't vary is this: to enter the zone of optimal performance, you must switch off the conscious mind.

Pressure Management Tools

Clearly, we need a strategy to avoid distraction, reframe the pressure of the moment, and focus on the task at hand. The following suggestions can help with this:

- Ground and center yourself to access and maintain the best state of mind for the task
- Remember past successes in similar situations, to boost confidence and tap into the same mindset used then
- See the pressure as a challenge or opportunity, giving things a positive rather than negative spin
- Visualize a successful outcome, which activates new neural pathways and helps maintain a positive state of mind
- Consider every situation a chance to improve, rather than a once-in-a-lifetime opportunity; this reduces overall stress during the performance
- Focus on what you can control in the moment
- Use a mantra to stay grounded and centered; this acts as a cue to anchor your focus and physiology
- Train in pressure situations, as often as possible; anticipate challenges and problems
- Do the best that you can in the moment; you don't have to break your personal record every time
- Use the ROADMAP System® for Performing Under Pressure (See Chapter 7).

One technique is to squeeze a ball in your left hand while repeating your mantra just before your performance. Squeezing the ball in your left hand primes the right hemisphere of the brain, which is associated with the subconscious neural pathways used for automatic skills. Activation of the right hemisphere also tones down left-hemisphere thoughts about success and failure.

Success Insurance for Choking, Sandbagging, Self-Handicapping, and Burnout

You can't think and hit at the same time.
Yogi Berra

How can you learn to optimize your performance, especially when the stakes are high? And what can we learn from those who fail under pressure in athletic, business, and other situations?

Cognitive neuroscientists and sports psychologists have studied performance under pressure, seeking to learn why some people do their best—and others their worst—when it matters the most. The four most common success completion problems are choking, sandbagging, self-handicapping, and burnout. Each of these issues can be overcome with a specific strategy.

Choking

When Jackie Robinson grabbed his throat after umpire Bill Stewart badly missed a call in a game between the Cardinals and the Dodgers, Stewart threw him out of the game. Choking became a common term for blowing it. Choking usually refers to failing at something under pressure, when you do that same thing well under other circumstances.

Some common choking scenarios:

- Botching a routine behavior, like catching a ball in a big game.
- Flubbing a well-practiced presentation.
- An actor forgetting lines he's said a hundred times before.
- Blanking on the name of someone the person knows quite well.

When any performer instantly shifts from the bottom-up to the top-down system – to think even for a second about technique, stepwise execution, or to try to ensure against a mistake – this dramatically alters the outcome of flow and performance, athletic and intellectual.

Three behaviors increase pressure:

1. Framing a situation as a unique experience:
    - This is my most important performance.
    - There will never be another opportunity like this.
    - Today I make history.

Thinking of a pressure moment as a single shot heightens the sense of risk and potential loss. With athletes, for example, loss aversion creates a behavior of playing "not to lose" rather than "playing to win."

In the 2017 American League baseball championships, Charlie Morton was the starting Astros pitcher in Game 3 against the Yankees. When he was interviewed before the game, he said, "This is the biggest game of my life." My response, as an Astros fan, was "Uh-oh."

The Yankees got six runs in the first two innings.

See how right my grandmother was? If you're not having fun, you're not doing it right.

2. Exaggerating a situation by:
    - Becoming too attached to the outcome.
    - Intensifying thoughts of fear and anxiety and focusing on failure versus success.
    - Shifting state due to anxiety, resulting in loss of focus and working memory.

3. Thinking too much:
    - My childhood hero was Mickey Mantle. The first thing I looked for in the daily paper (and the only thing I read other than "Dear Abby") was his statistical summary. I recall telling my parents how mad I was at them for not naming me "Mickey." I envisioned becoming a professional baseball player more than I did being a doctor, but I had the same difficulty as Michael Jordan with the curve ball.
    - In one interview, Mantle spoke of discussing batting tips with Ted Williams. Mantle was young at the time, and felt honored to be talking to Williams, who was the greatest batter in baseball history. Williams went into detail about hand position, grip, which hand leads in batting left and batting right. Mantle recalled the overwhelming but helpful detail of this mentoring. "I was thinking so much about this

> that I went 0-30 my next at-bats," he said. Overthinking is a kind of choke that can derail a performance at any level.

Why do some people perform at their best when the stakes are highest, and others at their worst?

Since the meaning we give to any event determines our response, changing the way we view anxiety and pressure can change their negative impact on performance. Regulating our state of mind is crucial. In fact, the greatest challenge in high-stakes performance is maintaining that performance mindset consistently in the face of various emotional triggers and charged situations, including extreme success.

In high-performance situations, the way you frame stress can significantly affect performance. Framing it as excitement and eagerness to perform is quite different than framing it as anxiety and fear of failure. And the actual performance often reflects this.

Pressure obviously increases anxiety but responding to this by paying too much attention to step-by-stop execution can make a smooth performance difficult or impossible. Worry requires mental energy that could otherwise be funneled into optimum performance. So, the more you worry about your performance, the less focus you have, and the worse your performance is likely to be.

For example, thinking about how someone else will react, or expecting to be criticized, can lead to a disruption in performance state of mind and flow, causing an inability to access crucial information that you already know quite well. Choking occurs when the focus shifts away from the performance for any reason. Sometimes this shift isn't even conscious.

Stereotypical triggers can also affect performance. For example, studies have shown that women perform worse on math tests when they are reminded of their gender beforehand. Race, ethnicity, and gender can all frame an unconscious bias. That bias can go either way, helping or hurting. This has nothing to do with ability, and everything to do with mindset.

In high-pressure situations, the ability to remain focused and in-state is everything. For example, in research examining 185 venture capital pitches, variables such as calmness, passion, eye contact and confidence were greater predictors of outcome than pitch content, experience, and expertise. The best outcomes went to those who maintained a state of confidence throughout.

Choking is not simply poor performance but failing to sustain what you're capable of. Trying to disregard, counter, or ignore a negative thought uses up valuable cognitive resources. Focusing on the task or performance at hand simplifies things and eliminates distractions.

At one point, tennis great Jana Novotna was a single point away from a Wimbledon championship victory over Steffi Graf. Under the pressure of competition (as she later explained), Jana began thinking about her next shot. This distraction resulted in double fault on her serves, and missed overhead shots played more cautiously than they should have been. Which caused her to lose the championship to Graf.

A remedy for choking: Remain in a flow state; do not shift to an observer state. This is true in all performance endeavors including sports, business, and the arts.

Advice drawn from research on sustained peak performance includes the following:

- Don't slow down. Any conscious thought about the process of control can compromise the flow state, resulting in loss of control.
- Practice under pressure. Simulate (as best you can) the exact conditions of the important performance. This trains mindset and execution and creates a hardwired path to success.
- Avoid distraction and dwelling on past failures. Reframe missteps as learning experiences.
- Use a key word as a cue to create and sustain focus throughout the performance: a single word that that represents successful mindset and execution.
- Focus on a positive outcome, rather than specifics of execution.
- Focus on what to do (the process) rather than how to do it (the technique).

A Specific Choke: the 'Yips'

The sudden inability to perform a basic, well-practiced skill—termed the yips by professional golfers (who experienced sudden tremors or jerks when trying to putt)—is found in every performance arena from sports to surgery. In shooting sports and archery, it's called target panic. In gymnastics and diving, balking. In competitive darts, it's dartitis. And for baseball pitchers, it's called

Steve Blass disease. It's a specific kind of "choke" of a motor function.

Pittsburgh Pirates starting pitcher Steve Blass suddenly lost his ability to pitch accurately. New York Yankees second baseman Chuck Knoblauch abruptly developed an incapacity to throw to first base. The common denominator was the derailed execution of a well-developed skill under pressure. In every case, the mental state change—which takes the player outside the performance zone—is the cause. Relaxation techniques, mental imagery, focus concentration and pressure management have proven ineffective in resolving such "performance blockages."

The content focus, whether it is the performance compromise, negative self-talk, or thinking about a component of the performance, instantly follows a shift away from the state of mind housing the peak performance skill. Analysis of components will not work, but will only sustain the altered state, disrupting the performance mindset and process.

Often, these performance inhibitions are due to some sports-related traumatic stress that have been identified in terms of origin but not corrected in terms of practice. The trauma could be an abusive coach, witnessing a fellow athlete's injury, or being injured oneself. These experiences become encapsulated in a particular state of mind—a time capsule that contains the fused trauma and inhibition. An emotional trigger or a specific performance cue/gesture can trigger an instantaneous entry into this time capsule and the immediate performance inhibition. Usual approaches combine some aspect of conscious focus and logical approaches to the issue, but the contents of that time capsule are not amenable to logic, reason, intellect, therapy, or reframing approaches. The time capsule houses the state of mind that originally experienced the trauma, a mind/brain/body combined experience.

The usual approaches to this issue ignore the fact that emotional memories are not amenable to logic, reason, intellect, or therapy.

Ken, a rising star catcher, was about to be called up any day to his major league baseball team roster. But he suddenly developed throwing difficulties. He had no trouble with the instant, automatic throws for a stealing base runner or rapid-fire play sequences. His difficulty was the simple throwback to the pitcher after each pitched ball. It was as if he had forgotten how to do a basic move he'd been practicing since the age of four.

This sudden onset of dysfunction occurred just after he took a forearm hit from a foul tip. It hurt for a while, but such things were routine, and he moved on—or seemed to. Somehow, though, the incident caused him to think about his throwing arm just after that inning. He noticed that he had errant throws going high, low, and wide. He was replaced before the end of the inning.

When the ball hit his forearm, it triggered memories of other physical injuries he'd experienced: a broken ankle in football, several jammed fingers, a broken index finger in baseball, and a hip bruise from a fastball. The new injury instantly booted up memories of those old sports injuries and the trauma that surrounded them.

We explored the frame-by-frame experience in his mind and found that the problem occurred when his routine throwing allowed him an instant to think about what he was doing. Yogi Berra's admonition that "You can't think and hit at the same time" certainly applied to Ken; he couldn't think and throw at the same time.

The team assumed it was an injury and put Ken on injured reserve status. But he knew the problem was in his mind, and that he needed to figure out a way to overcome it. He'd played through injury and pain before and managed to put those traumas behind him. But this one resonated with and activated this entire mindset. Each time he began a routine throwback to the pitcher, an instantaneous (and previously unconscious) association occurred that moved him away from the automatic skill he'd developed over two decades of practice into this time capsule of trauma.

Ken needed to stay in his performance mindset and avoid getting triggered into those traumatic memories. He developed a mantra that included a cue, a focus word, and a deep breath—and used the combination to sustain his performance state. He coupled the experience of gripping the ball with his focus word powerful and took a deep breath to draw relaxation in and push tension out. He repeated this scores of times each day, anchoring his ball-grip to an automatic performance state. Within ten days, he was throwing consistently and effortlessly.

When a choke occurs, look for the specific trigger that instantly recalls the traumatic experience that derails the performance.

Negative self-talk, a focusing on problems, and fear of performance all trace back to that memory-trigger. "Trying harder" and "practicing more" may only serve to reinforce the trigger. Rather than trying to "fix" every trauma-memory, we need to create an alternate pathway in the mind, one that points the trigger somewhere else. In this way, the trigger leads not to the old traumatic loop, but to the mindset and performance we desire. The Neural Conditioning Chart (Chapter 6) provides a map to help address these issues.

Self-Handicaps

Dr. Eddie O'Connor realized that when he failed to reach his running goal of completing a half mile in 2:10, he was holding back to have something left at the end of the race. He also hoped to reach the goal by "trying harder" next time. Eventually, he concluded that preserving the hope of "doing better next time" was interfering with his ability to do better now.

Self-handicaps are performance barriers or inhibitions created to attempt to protect someone's sense of confidence and self-esteem. Self-talk blames failures not on poor ability or preparation, but on some outside circumstance. This preserves the hope that one can do better by trying harder next time.

A remedy for self-handicaps: Self-reflection and awareness of the situation, so the performance flow state can resume.

Sandbagging

Sandbagging is designed to lower the pressure of performance anxiety by attempting to demonstrate a limitation or negative aspect to diminish others' expectations of you. Paradoxically, this also reduces the actual performance quality. In one study, sandbaggers who predicted lesser performances found themselves mired in self-fulfilling prophecies: “I may have lost, but it really doesn’t count, because I didn’t try.”

A slight variation of this may involve self-deception about your performance and obsessing over growth and excellence themselves. But playing for the sake of excellence is not all there is to sports or business.

Both self-handicapping and sandbagging are designed to preserve integrity and avert pain, yet both produce the very results they try to avoid. In either case, honest self-reflection can lead to a successful resolution. Self-reflection is a key component of recognizing, owning—and deciding what to change about—any aspect of performance.

A remedy for sandbagging: Change your self-talk to frame focus on performance challenge.

Burnout

A client I’ll call Evelyn consulted me about career burnout. She’d enjoyed remarkable and rapid success as an actress, moving quickly through local theater productions and national commercials to an award-winning role on a national series. Her energy brightened a room, induced optimism in others, and people were impressed with her imaginative and creative presence.

She was highly intuitive and sensitive, which made it easy for her to connect with others, and with the characters she played. But she also found herself unusually sensitive to the stressful emotions of those around her. This caused her to feel emotionally drained by crowds, and even by family, friends, and fans who approached her in public, seeking autographs or selfies with her. While Evelyn enjoyed her popularity and wanted to please people, she often felt depleted. She questioned whether this burnout meant she was unsuited for the job she loved.

We explored her state of mind she found herself in when feeling drained. She said she had to go home and felt depleted for hours. Naps failed to restore her energy. Her high degree of creativity and imagination made her a natural for her chosen work, but she lacked the necessary buffers and boundaries to regulate her state of mind, even in her private time. Evelyn needed an internal point of reference anchored in her own needs and ideals.

We focused on her need to remain grounded in her own experience. She developed a way to carve out private space and time for her own needs, and to establish boundaries when interacting with others. For example, she developed an awareness of how any character she inhabited for a screen role was itself a state of mind. She learned how to effectively enter and exit that state of mind every day, so she didn't take her work (and mindset) home with her. Evelyn needed to sustain her internal point of reference even more than most individuals, as her intuitive empathic style, at times selfless, was eroding the joy from her accomplishments.

She learned to limit her exposure to others and reduce the excessive stimulation of crowds and needy/negative people—all without feeling guilty for saying "no." She scheduled quiet time for emotional decompression and recharge, and learned the value of meditation. She took calming mini-breaks throughout the day and doing two-minute mindfulness meditations instead of yielding to reactive triggers. These practical strategies allowed her to conserve her energy and spend it on things she consciously chose. I also had her read *The Giving Tree* by Shel Silverstein.

In this book, a small boy approaches the tree to ask for help. The tree empathically listens to each need he has. Each need is compelling, so she gives him her apples to sell, her branches for a house, her trunk for his boat. She ultimately gives so much of herself—without regard to her own needs—that she is a stump, no longer able to sustain life.

By protecting herself in this way and being attuned to the necessary boundaries between herself and others, Evelyn was able to maintain her treasured sensitivity without becoming overwhelmed by her contact with others. A very visual person, her mantra included a visual focus instead of a word. She pictured herself surrounded by a cone of warm white light that offered energy and protection from negativity.

These necessary steps kept Evelyn centered in an otherwise very demanding world of fame, allowing her to sustain her energy and to fully contribute in ways that she valued. By more effectively grounding and centering herself and cultivating mindfulness, she developed a greater resilience to vulnerability of influence and emotions of others—and stopped placing the needs of others before their own. Her career soared even higher.

Burnout is a syndrome with symptoms including diminished emotional drive, concentration, motivation and enthusiasm for the endeavor at hand. Often the result of chronically stressful performances, burnout causes tension and fatigue, with decreased passion and consistency. Not surprisingly, various studies associate greater mindfulness with more positive engagement and a reduction in stress, exhaustion, and negativity.

Burnout may be the antithesis of resilience. A recent study of pediatrics residents (physicians) at Seattle Children's Hospital by Dr. Maneesh Barta found a burnout rate ranging from 41 to 77 percent, depending on the year of residency. Other studies show similar rates for other medical specialties. And higher burnout rates are associated with a higher incidence of medical errors.

A resilience training program was developed by the Mattel Children's Hospital Pediatric Residency at the David Geffen School of Medicine at UCLA. The findings uncovered some successful coping strategies:

- In an emotionally challenging situation, focus on possibilities rather than problems.
- When confronted with distraught individuals or an overwhelming personal emotional response, call a time-out to regulate your state of mind and restore balance.
- Plan best responses for situations that have no existing precedent or response template.
- Deeply inhale relaxation and exhale any tension.

Regulation and self-care are cornerstones of personal health and balance and enables the practitioner to better care for others. The secondary trauma experienced by caregivers can be as severe as that experienced by the victim.

A remedy for burnout: Mindfulness with reappraisal, reframing, and reengagement.

Chapter 10. The Art and Neuroscience of Winning

Forty-five minutes or so before the start, I'm not thinking about how to ski fast or what it takes to execute the perfect biathlon shot or how much a biathlon race hurts. I tell myself it's just skiing and it's just shooting, and I know how to do both of those things well. I ski through it in my mind, and I try to visualize what type of emotions I'm going to feel, what type of pressure I'm going to feel, before it actually happens. I'm thinking about the race. I'm thinking about where I'm going to change my technique, if it's slow snow, if it's fast snow, if it's windy, if it's not windy. In my mind I can see the changing of the digital numbers and for a moment I think, Can I do this? Am I capable of putting myself through this again? Usually, the crowd is screaming. It's pandemonium. But for me, that's the point where the audio and visual come in and become sort of a tunnel where the only thing that I'm focusing on is my own race, and in that moment, I have to repeat to myself, Do what you can with what you have where you are. That's Teddy Roosevelt's quote: "Do what you can, with what you have, where you are." A song comes on that distracts you for a second and it's all about getting back into your own zone, and for me that reset button is just repeating that quote. I look at the snow, I look at where I am. I've got skis on my feet. I've got a rifle on my back. I know how to start the race. I just need to let my body do it. I know that at ten seconds I'll hear the audible beeps and that's the trigger. I'm the bow with the arrow drawn waiting, and when that beep changes, that's the release and that's the acceleration and I'm the arrow and I'm accelerating down the track. Do what you can, with what you have, where you are.

From: "Inside the Mind of an Olympic Athlete Ten Minutes Before the Biathlon Race"

Lowell Bailey/Biathlon Olympic Event

Experts and Amateurs

When ya get to the end zone, act like ya been there before.

Coach Bum Phillips to rookie running back Earl Campbell

An expert and an amateur are each states of mind. "The expert" is an ideal, a contrast to "the amateur." Evolution from amateur to expert is a significant, life-changing passage when it occurs. The following distinctions can apply to that process of transformation.

Experts continue concentrated, deliberate practice on focused areas and develop with informed feedback.

Amateurs get to a level of good enough and stay there.

Experts seek practice and goals that exceed current levels of performance.

Amateurs seek to sustain a comfort level without challenging it.

Experts understand that there is no predetermined limit of ability.

Amateurs believe there is a fixed reserve of potential.

The expert works from love, passion, and dedication; failure is information to guide redirection and proceeding.

The amateur may be sidetracked by setback; failure is validation that he or she should not proceed.

The expert loves and pursues the game, whatever the game is, with total dedication and passion.

The amateur pursues it as a sideline, part time, like a weekend warrior.

The expert keeps going, no matter what.

The amateur is dissuaded by setback and adversity.

The expert does what is important first.

Amateurs do what is urgent first. Sometimes a football team can do more in the final two minutes of a half than in the previous twenty-eight, with little time remaining can focus energy, attention, and concentration. The expert operates for the entire game in this zone. The amateur waits for the two-minute warning.

An expert takes an initial step or performance cue to move toward the goal each practice, each day.

An amateur practices or performs when motivated.

The expert is on a mission, knows that fear can never be overcome, and recognizes that the best indication of what's next may be what generates the most fear. The expert knows that once action has begun, fear will recede, like your lap when you get up to walk.

The amateur must first overcome the fear, believing that comfortable is a prerequisite of beginning.

The expert knows that "fairness" is a childhood wish, that in adulthood there is not even an ultimate arbiter of fair. There is always adversity, unlevel fields, bad hops, rotten calls, injustice, unfairness.

The amateur seeks fairness and is set back by what does not seem fair.

The expert does whatever it takes, even for what never could have been imagined.

The amateur needs predictability, consistency, assuredness of results.

The expert respects the craft but is not superior to it, recognizing the contribution of those who have gone before, and are now alongside.

The amateur believes in inherent luck and intelligence and waits for inspiration to come.

The expert dedicates to mastery.

The amateur dedicates to proving himself or herself, needing to consistently demonstrate superiority and competence.

The expert does not take things or people personally, recognizes that others always make self-statements, and does not succumb to criticism, envy, or idealization of others.

The amateur is subject to the perception of others, to rejection, and reads the responses of others as if looking into an accurate mirror of a valid reflection.

The expert self-regulates and self-validates to take in new information but does not let it determine meaning.

The amateur becomes an extension of the interest, desire, and needs of others with vulnerable reliance on the perception and feedback of others.

The expert has an internal point of reference and is proactive.

The amateur has an external point of reference and is reactive.

The expert seeks the mastery of art as work, deliberate practice as lifestyle, success as creation.

The amateur believes that art is inspiration, talent is innate and seeks the lucky break.

The expert believes that the architect of magic is informed persistence and dedicated resilience.

The amateur believes that magic is magic.

The expert shows up every day, no matter what, and is committed for the long haul. The expert understands delayed gratification; is the ant, not the grasshopper; the tortoise, not the hare.

The amateur shows up as long as something else doesn't get in the way. The amateur looks for shortcuts, quick results, and immediate gratification.

Experts know they can do best that which they do uniquely well.

Amateurs try to do many things, to be everything to many people.

The expert always treats practice like a game.

The amateur saves the best for an actual game.

The expert knows that the self and every story line in life are created moment by moment, that the ultimate abandonment is of oneself.

The amateur believes that much is predetermined, some fate, some circumstance, some luck; that consistent attention must be received to be appreciated or accepted by others.

The expert believes that we write, live, and create in order to know.

The amateur believes that we must know in order to write, live, and create.

Experts add value to their art, to their science, to their expert body of knowledge, and to others.

Amateurs add value to themselves.

The expert believes that certainty develops with proceeding and mastery.

The amateur must have certainty to proceed.

The expert has a commitment and sticks to it no matter what.

The amateur responds to the prevailing mood, mindset, or urgency rather than purpose.

The expert, even at times a warrior, believes in humility and modesty.

The amateur believes in never showing vulnerability, doubt, or uncertainty.

The expert punches through the bag and runs through the finish line.

The amateur hits the front of the bag and relaxes at the finish line.

The expert knows that courage is to proceed despite fear.

The amateur believes that courage is the absence of fear.

The expert sticks to the plan.

The amateur lets life get in the way.

The expert determines what is important and works toward a purpose.

The amateur reacts to the urgencies of life.

The expert pursues the plan and purpose no matter how they feel.

The amateur acts when in the right mood or feeling.

The expert consistently pursues success despite a routine practice that might entail boredom.

The amateur pursues success when motivated or inspired.

Optimal Winning Performance: The Essentials

How do the best athletes/actors/executives become the best? And stay the best?

In a broad series of studies, performers experienced competition as more stressful than rehearsal or practice. Japanese researcher Michiko Yoshie investigated numerous professional pianists in practice and during competition to find that most pianists played worse in contests than in rehearsal and that it is rare to find someone who performs as well in competition as in practice. The winners were distinguished by one overarching factor: they performed as well in competition as they did in rehearsal.

Regulation of state of mind affects underlying physiology to regulate noradrenaline and adrenaline output, the two chemicals that mediate the physiological experience of stress. The physiological effects of performance anxiety can be modulated by method and strategy.

Mindfulness and pressure management tools directly affect training of the amygdala and the anterior cingulate cortex to regulate reaction to a mistake. Practiced focus to remain centered can sustain the relaxed focus characterized by the brain's alpha waves. Conscious slow breathing and specific focus regulate heart rate and stress response to avert beta waves prompted by anxiety.

Optimal regulation is not too much, not too little. Not too much in the sense of regulation to stress response, and not too little for an optimum level of arousal.

Self-regulation is the route to peak performance for most people. There are well-known exceptions to this, such as karate competitions and military operations in which anger can fuel a more optimal response. But those appear to be the exception.

Cortisol, usually synonymous with stress, weakens the immune system and hampers learning. Yet for successful competitors, the right amount of an increase in cortisol actually manages stress to enhance optimum performance. Cortisol regulates an enzyme that converts noradrenaline into adrenaline, improving the optimal balance between the two hormones.

Another hormone of competition is oxytocin, known to be the hormone of connection and bonding. Highest for a period of time during childbirth and at orgasm, it can create an intense competition when framed in this way of connection.

In the film The Blind Side, Michael Oher, although huge, gets pushed around by defenders and has difficulty blocking people to protect his quarterback. His adoptive mother pulls him aside to remind him how he ferociously protected his younger stepbrother and her in a bad part of town. She reminded him that the team is his family and that the quarterback can be thought of as her and how he had her back. She reminded him to think about how he would never let anything, or anyone hurt his little stepbrother or her. Tapping into these protective instincts unleashed oxytocin to fuel his protection of the blind side of his quarterback all the way through to the NFL. Whether in business or sports, relationships are paramount.

The vagus nerve is one of the pathways the brain and body use to talk to each other in unconscious conversation. Much of that conversation is about how we relate to others, tracking social engagement, connection, and cooperation.

A welcoming situation or engaging conversation greenlights brain and body to prepare for a positive, friendly engagement. The vagus nerve is a pathway mediating the oxytocin system, the chemical of bonding and connection. It has been shown that the first few words of a conversation can boot up this response, or, alternatively, if the perception is of a threat or a need for defense, the yellow light activates a fight/flight mode mediated by the neurochemical system of cortisol and adrenaline.

Can you try too hard?

Writer Lisa Cron noticed that when she misspelled a word, the more she tried to figure out how to spell it, the more mangled it became. She then noticed that if she quickly retyped it without thinking, most of the time she spelled it correctly. She concluded, facetiously, that her fingers know how to spell better than her brain.

In many cases we reduce accuracy by thinking too hard.

Nobel Laurate Herbert Simon believes that it takes roughly ten years to master a subject, the time it takes long-term conscious effort to develop expertise before the brain assigns it to the cognitive unconscious. It is at that point that many situations can be responded to intuitively, rapidly, and often without being able to specify the thinking sequence that led to a conclusion. At this point in the development of a finely honed skilled, we are no longer aware of the specific technical steps taken.

Andrew Campbell and colleagues studied why excellent leaders made bad decisions at particular times. He found two common elements: a current experience that elicited emotions that were tagged to past experiences, and prior response patterns that were superimposed on current responses.

Their findings relate to how instantaneous choices based on unconsciously coupled associations can be deconstructed to understand the components. The Neural Conditioning Program can be used to deconstruct an emotional trigger and understand the associated mindset. That content is like an old software program, with meanings, algorithms, associations, and content that will always be the same. Like a time capsule that is reentered. Trying to understand, resolve, or work through the issues of this altered state not only will be ineffective but will etch the groove of that state in your brain even further.

The proven success formula is to recognize the emotional triggers and the resulting state change—the process and the content of that state—to get grounded and centered to move immediately to an ideal response.

Playing to Win vs. Playing Not to Lose

Dominique Moceanu at age fourteen won an Olympic women's gymnastics gold medal in the 1996 Summer Olympics in Atlanta. It was the United States Olympic women's first-ever team gold medal. Moceanu appeared on magazine covers and talk shows after this remarkable feat.

But Moceanu peaked at the young age of fourteen, and instead of continuing a legacy four years later at the Sydney Olympics, she was the victim of unforced errors. She had burned out.

The reason for this burnout, as she later clearly articulated, was having a consistent external focus rather than a desire from within. She indicated that rather than an internal motivation and purposeful passion, she sought to avoid the authoritarian judgment and criticisms of her parents and coaches. "The sport I had loved so much was slowly becoming a nightmare as I trained with my coaches the summer before the [1996] Olympics," she said. "I pushed myself as hard as I could, but I always felt like I couldn't please them. As much as the coaches treated me with disdain and lack of respect, I kept trying to gain their approval. I feared Coach Bela Karolyi like I feared my father, Tata, yet I still tried to please both of them." After winning the gold medal in 1996, she was disappointed and did not celebrate with her teammates. "I realize then that no matter how much I wanted to feel happy, my happiness depended on what my coaches and parents thought of my performance and whether or not they were pleased with me," she said. "It was hard to be happy when I felt I wasn't perfect enough for them."

Her unforced errors came indirectly as a result of the fact that her point of reference was on pleasing others rather than an internal purpose and passion. Her fear of failure, which seemed to fuel her motivation at the time, became toxic. A fear of failure can lead, as it did with her, to stress, burnout, and diminished longevity.

For some competitors, competition facilitates creative output enhanced by motivation and effective preparation coupled with a comfort with conflict and opposition, a necessary building block for effective competition. Those whose performances suffer in competition, on the other hand, are intimidated by the intensity and emotionally withdraw.

How can framing of playing to win make a difference?

Rewards-driven behavior has an external point of reference and entails a drive to seek approval by others and external rewards. Being driven by fear means doing whatever it takes not to lose, to not disappoint others, and to focus only on results. Reframing fear as the excitement of achievement is a way to play to win rather than not to lose. The most fundamental distinction is this: if you focus on what you will win, you engage an optimum performance mindset.

We seek pleasure by playing to win. We avoid pain by playing not to lose. When you play not to lose, you most likely ensure loss because this shifts the operating system of the brain. The brain has two neurochemical systems, one wired to seek pleasure by winning, the other wired to curtail risk and avoid mistakes, to avoid pain and play not to lose. The two most fundamental motivations of seeking pleasure and avoiding pain are hardwired and supported by the software stories of our mind. Seeking pleasure leads to gain orientation, while avoiding pain leads to prevention orientation.

With gain orientation, we take risks and look for potential reward. This framing initiates an optimum performance mindset. Prevention orientation generates caution to avert risk. The closer we get to a goal, the greater the weight of the tendency to shift into prevention-orientation.

An application: a situation can be seen as a challenge—the perception of opportunity to shift mindset to the reward center to take risks, activating the gain-orientation system. A threat warns to shut down to avoid mistakes. Two very different mindsets with two different levels of performance and results. Most successful performance is in the challenge mindset.

In summary, some of the distinctions between playing to win and playing not to lose:

- Playing to win is based on confidence; playing not to lose is based on fear.
- Playing to win optimizes performance; playing not to lose is defensive.
- Playing to win is thriving and superiority; playing not to lose is surviving and mediocre.
- Playing to win creates special experiences and memories; playing not to lose creates stressful experience and moments.

- Playing to win optimizes abilities, playing not to lose compromises expression of abilities.

Shadow Stories of Competition and Performance

There are numerous games that people play in arenas and boardrooms in addition to the performance in which they are engaged. These games encompass a continuum of emotional responses, attitudes about winning and losing, motivations, and players' self-regard as participants.

Examples include the conscious focus of achieving excellence and the shadow story of proving oneself as good, worthy, or adequate. Other shadow stories involve achieving a personal perfection to appear competent to exceptional by others, to connect with others, to capture/recapture a youthful ideal, and even the more noble intent of the enjoyment of learning and skill acquisition. Doing well to deserve love and to be accepted by proving oneself may not be as far from the heart of the motivational orbit as we hope it would be.

If a measure of worth is based on how well you do in a performance, whatever it is, you become vulnerable and cannot disengage yourself from your perceived consequence of performance.

How we each interfere, sometimes significantly, with our ability to learn and perform becomes an important inquiry. We must learn about ourselves, our motivations, to learn how we best learn to discover our work and performance styles, personality components, and even and our biorhythms.

Can winning become a cultural or team identity?

The Hopi of Northwestern Arizona have inhabited a village, Oraibi for almost 1,000 years. The Hopi have more than a dozen ceremonial running races each fall. The Hopi women support the endeavor—and their identity—by phrases translating to "stay strong" and "dig deep" in Hopi language.

The men run several miles to their work in bean fields, past the graves of ancestors.

Hopi High has won 26 Arizona State Championships in a row, the longest in the country for cross-country races. Their coach, Juwan Nuvayokva, a former All American cross-country runner, captures this spirit and identity: "Hopi have that running blood in them. It's up to us to find it and use it." Hopi High is a school of 400 students in grade 9 through 12. Rick Baker, the Hopi High physical education teacher responsible for their cross-country program, said it simply, "A lot of our kids don't have a lot of speed. If you time them in the 400 meters they probably wouldn't break 70 seconds, but they have endurance. They can run and run and run."

The girls' team has won 22 state championships in 28 seasons. Their cultural identity was captured by a 70-year-old Hopi, Lee Grover, who said simply, "We are gifted with this talent of running. It's something we should never let die."

Can a performance culture have negative impact and consequence?

In 2016 an extensive scandal was exposed at Wells Fargo in which thousands of employees engaged in secretly creating new bank and credit card accounts for customers without their knowledge. Fake accounts with real customer money were so widespread at the bank that 5,300 Wells Fargo employees were fired over the issue. The Wells Fargo widespread employee cheating scandal led to a $185 million fine imposed by federal regulators. Thousands of branch employees secretly opened more than two million deposits or credit card accounts for customers who never asked for them. The number of employees involved and the length of time – five years – for this deception was remarkable.

The Wells Fargo scandal was different, partly in its magnitude, in that it was not a select few doing bad things, but tens of thousands of employees engaged in secretly defrauding customers resulting in overdraft and other fees.

Wells Fargo had aggressive goals coupled with performance pressure and with stretch objectives that generated social contagion impacting employees' ethics. One former Wells Fargo branch manager told the Los Angeles Times, "We were constantly told we would end up working for McDonald's if we did not make the sales quotas… We had to stay for what felt like an afterschool detention, or report to a call session on Saturdays." It was reported that inside the banking system, the attitude was, "Do what you have to do but don't get caught." "All the tellers knew of the frauds, but… people needed the job." When pressured, they opted for self-protection as a survival mode in the face of pressure, and their ethics dissolved in the process.

Cheating is fostered by both performance pressure and group culture. The pressure to outperform can then make cheating feel justified. Dan Ariely has studied this behavior and found two conditions that increase cheating behavior:

- A social environment where you see cheating around you
- The more people are removed from actual money. More abstraction involves dealing with derivatives such as the complex instruments Madoff and Stanford dealt with that even other money managers said they didn't understand. Ponzi used the arbitrage of international reply coupons for postage stamps, also very little understood at the time.

Rationalization can bypass personal values, judgment, and ethics. A business mindset of "it's just business" categorically justifies behavior that may be dishonest or lacking morality by focusing on the commercial aspect.

Chapter 11. Achievement and Success: Mastering the Extremes

Fame has killed more very talented guys than drugs.
Keith Richards

Exceptional Achievement and Overconfidence

It was very difficult to see him become even bigger than life. He had so much so soon. He was snatched from the ordinary life of a young man into a place that no one had ever been in society or in our culture.
Priscilla Presley on Elvis Presley

Ask any player in a physician's basketball league whether they can compete with LeBron James, and they'll laugh. Yet many of those same physicians willingly compete with the billionaire investor Warren Buffett. Cognitive biases and mental errors make them believe they can outperform successful full-time investment experts with decades of experience.

Those who've achieved in exceptional ways can create challenges for themselves when it comes to managing their success. Some highly successful individuals, from actors and athletes to practicing medical and legal experts, begin to believe that they can excel in other areas, like investing. But expertise in one area seldom translates to expertise in another. Even Warren Buffett recognizes this about himself: "I don't think being able to allocate capital means you're good at anything else."

Overconfidence, fueled by spectacular success in one area, creates a misperception of overall ability. University of Pennsylvania psychologists Phillip Tetlock and Barbara Mellers studied more than twenty-five thousand forecasts from people whose task was to anticipate how the future would unfold. Their studies, like several others, revealed exceptional overconfidence from successful doctors, lawyers, engineers and even scientists.

From Macbeth we learn that we are most vulnerable not when we are beginning, or even when destitute or needy, but after the biggest triumphs of our lives. For Macbeth, the moment the witches came just after he won his two greatest battles and was enjoying immense popularity.

The stimulation of overconfidence is biologically habituating. Look at the lessons from politicians, actors, and athletes who came to believe that their success made them immune to boundary violations: Elvis, Marilyn, Janis, F. Scott, Kurt, Belushi, and Philip Seymour among others. *Some people need mentor coaches not to become successful, but to help them regulate their states of mind and manage their emotions to sustain success.*

Exceptional success can elevate the individual beyond expectations, as when an athlete breaks records, or when accomplishments in other fields exceed any possible preparation. Such situations create unique challenges.

A significant factor in performance psychology is that excellence is not normal. The top 1% do what the other 99% are unable or unwilling to do. The pursuit of excellence and expertise requires dedication and resilience.

The more we know and the better we become, the more likely we are to overestimate our own abilities, and to underestimate the events beyond our control. In one study, CEOs became more confident as they gained merger and acquisition experience, which led them to overvalue subsequent deals. In research from the University of Vienna, investors who obtained significant experience with their market became overconfident and tended to engage in risky asset trades.

Assessing overconfidence becomes a challenge. We strive to make confidence a state of mind, but when the process becomes subconscious (as it should), omissions of logic are hard to detect. Confidence can generate remarkable productivity, but overconfidence can bring it all crashing down.

Overconfidence grows with sustained success and power and can replace self-reflection with blind certainty. Overconfidence increases with familiarity, repetition and continued success. One of the best predictors of overconfidence is power, which can lead one to overlook necessary questions and alternate paths.

The more any action is rewarded, the quicker it becomes a habit, and the harder it is to break. After a while, habits become automated; a default mode that we don't even think about.

Can success itself become intoxicating?

The boiling frog metaphor is a caution against the gradual and unknowing acceptance of change. Escalating success can cause other values and ideals (like family) to fall by the wayside. Sacrifice (in pursuit of excellence) can become both justified and idealized.

The excited stimulation of success can become intoxicating, making it harder to regulate emotions and stay grounded in identity and ideals. This process can be gradual and unnoticed. Soon one considers oneself special, entitled, and immune from ordinary consequences. Success builds on itself and becomes seductive. The goal of "more" can create an intolerance of obstacles. And while "success intoxication" has no evil intent or motivation, the results can be destructive. Great accomplishments lead to a desire for still greater accomplishments, regardless of what it takes to get there.

Because the stimulation of achievement is invigorating, it may become harder to just relax. As success places greater demands on time and attention, boundaries between work and personal life may become blurred or eroded. Self-esteem can become exaggerated because of constant stimulation and feedback. The metrics of success need to continue to grow, just to maintain the same level of satisfaction and excitement. The whole thing can become like a drug habit.

It may take a personal or professional crisis to crystalize awareness of this process in the mind. Sometimes, people will unconsciously create a crisis in order just to step off the treadmill they feel powerless to stop.

How can extreme success be mastered and maintained?

The toughest thing about success is that you got to keep on being a success.
Irving Berlin

As Althea Gibson, winner of eleven major tennis titles and the first African American to be named "female athlete of the year" by WHO, has observed, "Most of us who aspire to be tops in our field don't really consider the amount of work required to stay tops." The relentless, repetitive work of deliberate practice is essential, and no less grueling to maintain at the top of one's field.

The two fundamental challenges that come after achieving remarkable success are:

1. How to sustain and expand it
2. How to deal with the accompanying results, like fame and money

How do you navigate something you've never experienced? What do you need to know next, and how can you find a trusted guide to the uncharted waters of unprecedented success?

A specific challenge for those who achieve extreme success is figuring out a way to stay passionate about the pursuit of excellence, rather than indulging the inevitable temptation to simply enjoy the fruits and bask in the glow.

Top performers are not distracted by the victories or failures of themselves or others. They focus on the areas where they can be effective and let go of everything else. They know that it is the task at hand that matters, including the flow of the performance endeavor. This exclusive focus, a type of compartmentalization, fuels resilient practice and sustained peak performance. Elite performers have learned to embrace the pressure and immerse themselves in the process.

Elite performers in business, sports, and the arts are often equally passionate about their hobbies. Richard Branson is as passionate about his hot air balloon adventures as he is about his primary business. Football player J.J. Watt became consumed in the offseason, helping Hurricane Harvey flood victims in Houston with a passion equal to that he brings to the game. Such intensely focused passion and purpose often imbues top performers with the ability to rebound from defeat

Teams and companies continually push one another to superb performance, achieving levels unattainable when working alone or with less-accomplished colleagues.

Outstanding new performers in every domain have an insatiable appetite for feedback to use in analysis, deliberate practice and performance. They celebrate their accomplishments, the celebration serving as reward and emotional release. A constant dialectic can balance continued striving and accomplishment with celebration.

How can a sense of purpose sustain success?

Like talent, purpose is not inherent or discovered but cultivated. Passion, purpose, and talent all need to be developed by deliberate effort and practice.

Several research findings reveal that individuals who have a strong sense of purpose are more willing to persist and take risks. They also have a significantly higher percentage of successful outcomes, regardless of their area of expertise.

It's imperative for a team to have a shared purpose to unite players in striving for optimum performance, both individually and collectively. Many studies of exceptional performance find that the outstanding performer can catalyze teammates to excel. The star performer can be either a distraction, or a motivator for excellence. Exceptional immunologists boosted their colleagues' research productivity by 35 percent; the most outstanding 6 percent of physicists led research teams that generated 50 percent of all physics papers published. Wharton School of Business Professor Adam Grant has shown in his research that when people see how their work affects others and have a shared purpose. They work better, harder, longer, more generously and more productively.

To make purpose come alive, the coach must engage players and make them understand how their efforts make a difference for each other and the team's greater good. Team motivation is enhanced by an appreciation of the way in which everyone's work benefits the well-being of others and the team as a whole.

How can gender, race, and socioeconomic biases affect performance?

High-stakes performances, from tests to games to presentations, can ratchet up stress levels to the point where they interfere with the maintenance of performance flow and continued optimum performance. Stress can reduce the cohesive functioning of different parts of the brain that must work together to achieve an optimum result.

Cognitive horsepower relies on the prefrontal cortex, which houses working memory. Stress alters the ways in which different parts of the brain communicate. The fluid functioning of all brain areas, working individually and in concert, produces maximum effectiveness. Just like a team. Also like a team, anything that interferes with one component, or hampers communication, can compromise results

Stress can take many forms. A high stakes playoff performance. A woman who is the only representative of a race in a premiere doctoral program. The only Latino at an all-white firm. The only woman in an entire corporate division.

A study was done to see if the racial achievement gap could be mitigated or eliminated. A simple intervention resulted in a far greater change than the research group had ever imagined. Cohen and his colleagues found a middle school with a student population of roughly 50% African American and 50% white kids, with a significant classroom performance gap between them.

The researchers asked the teachers to administer an exercise packet to all seventh graders. Each student randomly received one of two packets. The teachers couldn't tell, from the envelopes, which student received which packet, and the students didn't know they were part of a study.

Students in the intervention group were shown values, then asked to choose the one most important to them and write about why it was meaningful to them. Students in the control group were asked to pick the value least important to them and write about why it might be important to someone else, but not them.

At the end of the semester, over 70% of the black students in the treatment/intervention group (who wrote about their most significant personal value) performed significantly better. For white students, there was no difference between the two groups. This simple 15-minute exercise resulted in a 40% reduction in the racial achievement gap. The exercise was repeated a year later with different students, with the same results.

A temporary condition of *stereotype threat* can zap the performance effectiveness of an individual or group stereotyped as academically inferior. Other studies included female students in math and science courses, and Latino and African American students on tests of intellectual ability (after being made specifically aware of their ethnicity or gender as an initial framework). These studies, too, emphasize how mindset and framework can affect performance.

Success Anticlimax

To travel hopefully is a better thing than to arrive.
Robert Louis Stevenson

The morning after Bruce Jenner's last Decathlon at the Montreal Olympics, he asked, "What am I going to do now?"

Olympic gold medalist Victoria Pendleton offered a slightly more elaborate comment on the same dynamic. "People think it's hard when you lose," she observed.

"But it's almost easier to come in second because you have something to aim for when you finish. When you win, you suddenly feel lost."

I vividly recall my favorite athletic coach introducing me to his version of this issue. As a freshman, I was fortunate to make the traveling squad of 12 basketball players, even though I felt intimidated by the upperclassmen surrounding me. Just after we won our first tournament and boarded our bus, Coach stood up front and looked at us. We were all feeling pretty good about the big win and were eager to get home and celebrate with a parade downtown. "So, we won this tournament," Coach said. "This is not the biggest or the most prestigious tournament that we'll play. It's kind of a Podunk tournament." He paused. "How many of you can really say you're proud to win this tournament?" Under any other circumstances, I would have raised my hand—as I suspected every one of my teammates also wanted to, but no one dared venture a single finger in the air.

"Feel good for now," he said. "But let's get home and really start working on being an excellent team."

Coach knew how to handle success anticlimax. His coaching and mentoring were life-changing for me and led to many wins and several championships. More importantly, it also guided me toward my two professional careers to help others succeed.

For any successful physical or intellectual achievement, the emotional role and creative closure needs to be addressed for successful completion. I've known a number of authors who described a let-down after their books were completed. One even described it as a postpartum-like depression (and that was a guy). The most successful achievers evolve their capacities to recover faster from success anticlimax.

After a long-practiced and anticipated success, people often must deal with a significant anticlimax experience. The sprint system of anticipation is mediated by dopamine, a pleasure chemical that can sustain the excitement of expectation when we anticipate a positive consequence. This can last, as we know from various performers, for years or in some instances decades.

After a significant achievement, and the continued stimulation of new challenges and endeavors, reaching the summit of success sometimes has the paradoxical effect of diminishing motivation. The "buzz" may be missing; the continued dopamine stimulation of "what's next" is no longer there, because all the "next" challenges and opportunities have already been achieved.

With no new stimulation or challenge, the competitive edge can morph into boredom and lack of motivation. Common questions at this point include "Did I lose my edge?" and "What's left to achieve?" The novelty, challenge, and quest for the next big achievement during all the stages leading to the successful attainment are no longer there.

This is very different from "burnout," and the depletion caused by intolerable workloads. Instead, this anticlimax simply means that the framework of novelty and the challenge of climbing the mountain need to be reframed. This is necessary to sustain passion and maintain interest in staying at the top to exceed former visions and definitions of success.

Rather than indicating a plateau, this experience can be a signal to look for access to the next level of achievement, to reframe interest and challenge for an even higher level of performance. Knowing that the brain craves novelty, this reframe/challenge may involve something not previously envisioned or attempted.

A coach can be a catalyst, empowering others to produce extraordinary outcomes for individual players and the team as a whole. Transformational coaches look beyond immediate goals and shape larger strategies that help individuals and teams to continually evolve.

A successful performance achievement profile is not a single straight line to peak success, but a process of continued practice and performance, including ups and downs. Performers must be able to sustain and enhance achieved success—tasks made more difficult when achievements have exceeded initial expectations.

What makes super achievers in sports, arts, or business so relentless in their successes?

It's about squeezing every last ounce of juice out of this life. We'll celebrate some things, but we'll very, very quickly move on to what's next.

Andrew Garfield, Tony and Golden Globe Award-Winning Actor

Relentless super achievers have something far simpler than genes, training, education, or internal drive. The athletes and executives I've worked with (and others I've interviewed or studied) have learned how to contend with the anticlimax of success and sustain anticipation by laddering achievement to focus on what's next.

Sustained achievement involves dealing with anticlimax faster and more effectively to emotionally disengage from a long-sought goal—and refocus on new endeavors.

This attitude was succinctly summarized by Manchester United Soccer Club manager Sir Alex Ferguson. Just a few minutes after holding up a record ninth Premier League soccer trophy, he said, "I'm already looking forward to next season. Let's get on with it. I'm looking forward to going on to win a European Trophy as well as pushing for the league." The next year, they did just that.

The dual challenge of maintaining and extending extreme success means sustaining the passion for continued growth and navigating the unprecedented challenges that accompany success. Super achievers share the following qualities:

- Dedication to a vision, with consistent purpose and focus.
- Persistence in a growth mindset that incorporates self-reflection and accurate performance assessment.
- Use of feedback to make necessary course adjustments.
- Emotion management and self-regulation.
- Learning and adapting on the fly.
- A growth mindset that seeks improvement even after success.

Nick Saban, head football coach at the University of Alabama, consistently tells his players to not think about championships and wins, but about the preparation and the performance of the process itself, *every day in practice.*

Often the performer does not recognize or reflect on different stages of the performance trajectory/career or understand the entire process in terms of developmental stages. The winning formula that got them up the mountain becomes an outdated game plan, even a handicap, once they've reached the top. A different system and a different identity are required at this point, and that requires a new effort and internal model.

Self-regulation can be a challenge for someone like a very young athlete, who's suddenly paid millions (or tens of millions) of dollars, especially when coming from a life of low income or poverty. There's no adjustment period, no time to adapt.

When anyone engages a task or position that moves them beyond their core identity, discomfort and uncertainty follow. More than 80 percent of those who win lotteries of $3 million or more, declare bankruptcy within five years. Their money changed, but their mindset did not.

The Summit Syndrome

The arrogance of success is to think that what you did yesterday will be sufficient for tomorrow.
William Pollard

What causes a practice or performance stall?

A large study of North Carolina teachers showed that they improved significantly during their first two years of teaching experience. After that, most stalled. Teachers with 27 years of experience were barely more effective than those with two years, when measured by student achievement in English and math. After reaching a certain level of achievement and satisfaction, the tendency was to stop looking for ways to improve.

As skill and expertise develop, one challenge is to avoid such development plateaus, where progress appears to cease. Initially challenged to enhance skills and expertise, we tend—with regular practice—to go on "automatic pilot." And the moment a particular behavior becomes a default mode, learning stalls.

The remedy is to focus on deliberate practice; on what can be learned and improved. Top performers keep learning, improving, and performing in new and better ways. Researchers have found that those who continue to push boundaries—even when already successful—and continue deliberate practice, continue to grow. Magnus Carlsen found that 74% of the top performers in his study of chess players reviewed their work consistently to learn and improve. Only 17% of people in the underperforming category did that. Top performers never stop learning.

What can you do to sustain motivation in practice and training, even after significant success?

There are a lot of people in the world who will take the challenge to climb the mountain. But when you get to the top of the mountain, you become the mountain

because everybody's shooting at you. The great ones can get to the top of the mountain and say, "You know what, I can be even better."
HBO Sports: Belichick and Saban

We do what we do because we imagine how it will feel when we do it. Playing to win has a more powerful and sustaining motivation than playing not to lose (to avoid embarrassment or the bad feeling associated with a loss).

Motivation is not enough. Even a stellar goal is not enough. A common statement is, "I need to get motivated to lose weight/workout/save money." Motivation is not only insufficient, it's not even necessary. All that's needed is a plan, and a commitment to stick to it. When you want to change, create a system—a map—and commit to consistently follow it. There are two basic considerations here:

- What's the greater pain if you don't proceed?
- What's the greater pleasure if you do proceed?

The desire to be better at what you're doing may be the only incentive necessary for success. Motivation is not intrinsic; desire and pleasure-seeking are. Once you practice something and become good at it, the skill itself creates the experience of effectiveness, which then enhances the desire. Ultimately, a sense of identity evolves. This becomes a powerful organizer for what you do, and can significantly resemble motivation.

Make it easy. Two o'clock p.m. is when my energy biorhythm dips. It's not my most creative time and, left to my own devices, I'd take a 15-minute nap. Instead, I view it as the best time to work out—and I return energized and ready to go. I never schedule clients during this time; nothing interferes with my workout unless it's an emergency. I don't work out at 2:00 every afternoon because I'm motivated to work out. I did initially, because I created a schedule to do at that specific time, and stuck to it. Now I do it for a different reason: it's who I am. It's part of my identity to do it for mind, body, and spiritual wellness. If I don't do it, I've not lived up to my ideal of myself. And when I do it, it confirms who I am.

Those supercharged and successful performers who consistently acquire new knowledge and evolve new skills, surpass even their own previous benchmarks of excellence. They push their own limits and expand the expected and (at times) exceed their own visions. Their identity coalesces around challenge, resilience, and successful performance.

George Parsons and Richard Pascale offer an interesting perspective to my research on and work with performers who experience success anticlimax. They described the corporate equivalent in the Harvard Business Review, how "steps taken at the right time not only can allow extreme overachievers to surmount the summit syndrome but can also deepen their capacity to lead."

Throughout the process of deliberate practice and resulting success, performers generate a heightened appetite for stimulation. Unless this is planned for ahead of time—with an eye toward next actions—it can create a vulnerability to distracting substitutes like drugs, risky investments, and exciting but bad relationships. Often, the peak of career success, when the performer feels most invulnerable, is the very time when they are most *vulnerable*. This is particularly true when the performer attempts to recapture or replicate the stimulation of success in alternate (often destructive) ways.

At this point, internal and external may not match. The external metrics of immense success may be overwritten by habituation to success, to wondering about what's next, to being confused about how to sustain the achievement excitement.

This process is often found among professional athletes, after the sudden achievement of a lifelong goal (Bruce Jenner, for example), or the end of a career after injury or retirement. In such cases, self-regulation challenges occupy the foreground, ranging from the continued stimulation of "what's next?" to the perceived difficulty of sustaining excitement and drive after reaching the summit.

Challenge can be diminished or negated when the outcome is certain. This takes away the thrill of the dopamine-mediated stimulation that asks, "What's next?" Think about the major successes you've achieved, probably with sustained immersion and dedication—the outcome of which was not determined until the very end. Throughout, "What do I need to do next?" sustains attention and stimulation. Think about how different the experience might be, if you knew that everyone who participated would get the same trophy or reward. This is not the way the mind, brain, or life works.

Significant Success: Liberation vs. Catastrophe?

When he was in his twenties, Pablo Picasso outrageously drew a group of prostitutes in a brothel, with faces resembling primitive African masks, and dismembered cubic limbs. This leap of imagination was called Les Demoiselles d (Avignon). In 218 BC, the Carthaginian general Hannibal (then in his 20s) attacked the Roman Empire. Albert Einstein, also in his 20s, changed the way we see space, time, light, energy, and the universe. Remarkable success can create triumphant heroes, and open the potential for growth and continued unsurpassed accomplishment, for which there are no precedents or models.

Tennessee Williams, who continued with a growth mindset and produced many successful plays, wrote in The Glass Menagerie that, after a number of people become successful and the initial thrill wears off, they perceive their success as a catastrophe, even “a kind of death.” This paradox has been expressed by athletes, executives, scientists, entrepreneurs, generals, performers and politicians. This syndrome was captured by economist Paul Samuelson, winner of the Nobel Prize, when he said, “After winners receive the award and adulation, they wither away into vainglorious sterility.”

A key element—perhaps the key element—in dealing with extreme success is to sustain a growth mindset in an evolving way, to not only continue the initial success, but to self-regulate the extreme emotional components and challenges of dealing with the accompaniments and sequelae of that success. In Tennessee Williams’ essay, “The Catastrophe of Success” he details the experience of moving from virtual oblivion to sudden prominence after publication of The Glass Menagerie. He describes becoming aware of how much energy had gone into the struggle, only after the struggle was removed. He then felt suddenly depressed in the midst of his success and the accompanying monetary rewards. Williams writes of a spiritual dislocation and becoming indifferent to the people around him. Cynicism replaced sincerity and kindness, and he grew suspicious of friends who offered inane flattery. And he realized that as he became indifferent, he began to dislike praise because it made him concerned that, "I felt too lifeless inside to create another successful play."

Perhaps the most succinct observation along these lines was made by Kurt Vonnegut to his friend Joseph Heller at a party on Shelter Island, given by a billionaire hedge fund manager. Vonnegut noted that their host had made more money in a single day than Heller had earned from his bestseller *Catch-22* over its entire history. Heller responded, "Yes, but I have something he will never have – enough."

More, like perfect, has no end, and will therefore never be attained. When enough has no end, the pursuit becomes relentless and unsatisfied.

The Hedonic Treadmill

Wealth is like seawater; the more we drink, the thirstier we become; and the same is true of fame.
Arthur Schopenhauer, 19th Century Philosopher

Psychologist and Nobel Prizewinner Daniel Kahneman described the hedonic treadmill as an ever-escalating pursuit of success which ensures that present success is never quite enough. The adaptation to escalating success is a biological and psychological phenomenon of the mind and body's adaptation to the initial pleasure of dopamine, and the attempt to restore that initial experience. Inevitably, subsequent restoration by drug or deed inevitably falls a bit short. Any form of success activates this pattern of attempting to replicate the initial performance/money/fame etc. high, engaging in pursuit and running faster, but never quite arriving.

Social scientist Arthur Brooks suggests that the Rolling Stones' "(I Can't Get No) Satisfaction" should properly be titled "(I Can't Keep No) Satisfaction".

The rewards from the hedonic treadmill tend to be extrinsic rewards. True satisfaction may result more from managing desires than increasing attainments. The things that provide real individual meaning come from within: needs, ideals, and purpose.

The antithesis of the hedonic treadmill is a step-by-step, strategic focus on the system and not just the goals. Both winners and losers have the same goals. After achieving remarkable success, continuing with the system maintains and enhances that success. If the objective is to reach the goal, you're done when you reach it. Identity then transforms to include sustained, expanding success, not celebration or results.

Unforced Errors

I think self-awareness is probably the most important thing towards being a champion.
Billie Jean King

Perhaps one of the best self-reflections—although done in retrospect—comes from John McEnroe in his book *You Cannot Be Serious*: “For the first few years, I almost never spoke an obscenity to an umpire or linesman. Then, at a certain point, I went over the line. There were reasons for it—reasons, not excuses … Once I began to go over the line, I should have been defaulted [disqualified].”

He was not disqualified for his famously bad behavior on the tennis court because by that time he was a highly regarded superstar. At an earlier point in his career, however, and in the careers of less famous players, that same behavior would have constituted an unforced error. Publicly challenging a teammate or coach becomes indicates a failure to self-regulate and maintain the performance zone.

Unforced errors are self-generated and completely avoidable. Mistakes that can sabotage a performance or a reputation need to be studied as certainly as success factors and strategies. Dr. Leo Levin introduced the term *unforced error* in 1982, to describe as an error in tennis competition that is “committed without a cause.”

In tennis, the literal term refers to an error committed by someone who has every capacity to keep the ball in play, but makes a mistake not caused by the other person's play. Often the player who makes the fewest unforced errors wins.

Extreme success brings its own neural chemistry, mindset, and challenges. At times, a feeling of invincibility (and the often-accompanying self-indulgence) can increase the likelihood of unforced errors because of diminished objectivity.

Just as people seek outcomes that best gratify their preexisting biases and desires (labeled at times as purposeful choices), executives and coaches can always find a way to eliminate people they don't want or who don't fit their profile of beliefs. Positions are eliminated, players are cut, and employees are laid off.

Because unforced errors are not always conscious or logical, reflection becomes a crucial component of recognition and behavior revision. The most insidious and potentially dangerous errors are ones that arise from unconscious biases, inattention blindness, and other judgment calls that are not recognized by the person who makes them. Even if they were pointed out, the performer might double down on mistakes to compensate, defend or deny. A simple mistake is not an unforced error, but persistence, compensation, and defense of poor decisions in the face of contradictory evidence can create unforced errors.

Operating and Non-Operating Performance Errors

The first task is to recognize the type of unforced error and consider various perspectives to devise remedies for optimizing performance.

Jeffrey Krames identifies two types of serious unforced errors: the unforced operating error, and the less common unforced non-operating error. An unforced operating error happens when someone makes a wrong decision and sticks with it. The introduction of New Coke in 1985 by CEO Roberto Goizueta, and the pushing of SUVs by car manufacturers while gas prices were soaring would be examples of this.

An unforced non-operating error is the result of bad judgment regarding discipline, self-control or character, sexual misconduct with an employee, insider trading or other ethics violations, for example. Arrogance, a sense of entitlement, and the hubris of power can all lead to unforced operating errors.

Some unforced errors are not necessarily fixed and need not automatically result in reassignment or firing. Those individuals who are willing to honestly and objectively assess, understand, and address the reasons for their errors can engage successfully. The issues can be engaged within the strength of a resilient working alliance and in the coach's understanding of the necessary components for recognition and change. An important aspect is that the coach does not take it personally, fosters the best efforts of the player, and believes in the process of change.

One kind of unforced error is assuming that those higher up on the team chart know more than you do, coupled with a failure to seek information from people throughout the team (including those below you).

The Ultimate Unforced Error: Fatal Flaws

A focus on improving strengths (as opposed to an excessive focus on weaknesses) is the best overall strategy. Still, there are some weaknesses that cannot be ignored because they may turn out to be fatal flaws.

No amount of brilliance or peak performance can counter a truly fatal flaw. Such flaws include a spectrum of character issues like dishonesty, cheating, and lying.

On the other hand, some "fatal flaws" can be overcome with attention and strategy. It's best to catch such issues—and address them—early on. These include:

- An unwillingness to learn from mistakes. This is not simply the lack of a growth mindset but denying or hiding mistakes (which makes it impossible to learn and correct).
- A failure to consider alternatives. This is a maintenance of the default mode or status quo, while failing to consider new ideas or ways of doing things (thus halting progress).
- Failure to appreciate or develop the collaborative and interpersonal skills that help move any endeavor forward.
- Blaming others for problems and claiming credit for success when neither is accurate (which can demoralize the whole team)
- A passive rather that active outlook, which ensures that unforced error (when present) will continue.

Remedies for these unforced errors include considering alternatives, reflecting on strengths and weaknesses, seriously considering all feedback, making adjustments in performance, and keeping an open mind with a proactive growth mindset. Confronting and addressing weaknesses—to further develop strengths—helps create a solid foundation for growth.

Unforced Errors: When Passion Derails

The obsessive pursuit of a passionate endeavor can result in tunnel vision. One prominent example of this would be Elizabeth Holmes, founder and CEO of the biotech company Theranos. And her father worked with Jeffrey Skilling at Enron—itself a cautionary tale.

The federal government indicted both Skilling and Holmes for massive fraud. Theranos was at one point valued at $9 billion, and Skilling was CEO of a $60 billion company. Fortune magazine declared Enron the most innovative large corporation in America. By all known accounts, neither initially sought to defraud the public, and each had a relentless passion that may have blinded them to anything other than its total and obsessional pursuit.

Unforced errors are especially likely to occur when someone loses their enjoyment of the pursuit itself and focuses only on winning. Such errors are compounded when the success is so huge that there are no precedents or reference models.

Sometimes the performer's point of reference shifts from an internal one (associated with needs and ideals) to an external one (focused on rewards and accolades), to the point where even constantly escalating achievement never seems good enough. The rewards and their anticipation transcend the joy and supposed purpose of

the activity itself. If there is no clear and attainable internal ideal—no “good enough” to achieve—validation shifts to an external source.

Relying on the opinions of others to determine how you feel about yourself, creates an immediate vulnerability and a framework of ineffectiveness, because no one can ever respond exactly as you script them to. External validation seems rewarding in the short term, but the ever ascending and never-ending desire for more is always there. And when someone fails to act as though they’re a simple extension of your interest or desire, frustration and ineffectiveness result.

Continuing success can also be threatened or derailed by performance-enhancing drugs, plagiarism, cheating and other unethical behaviors.

Success can also be squandered by *self-defeating attitudes* like:

- It’s too good to be true.
- Something’s bound to happen.
- This can’t last.
- The other shoe will drop.
- When something good happens, I don’t want to be surprised, so I get ready for bad things to happen.
- I expect the worst, so if it happens, I’m ready; if not, I’m surprised.

Or *self-destructive thoughts* like:

- I’ll beat disappointment to the punch (which ensures disappointment).
- I’ll rehearse a disappointment (which creates its enactment).

- If I give in to joy, I'll set myself up for disappointment.
- If I'm satisfied with "enough," I'll lose my motivation for more.
- Nothing will ever be enough, so why go all out?
- I'll push the bad image or behavior cue out of my head (which makes it more likely).
- I'll focus on the negative to avoid it (which gives it energy).

Extreme success creates a potential vulnerability simply because it transcends familiar experiences and known models. One way to end the discomfort caused by such an unfamiliar situation is to go back to the familiar—which will end the discomfort but forfeit the pursuit of excellence.

A ROADMAP System for Unforced Errors

Recognize that you are making an error.

> Otherwise, you'll fail to take corrective action and will keep making the same error.

Own the responsibility for committing the error.

> And for whatever impacts the error creates. Factors may include a failure to incorporate feedback or other relevant information. The performer is not always aware of errors at the time they're made. Admitting to them is the first step toward their elimination—and toward ever-greater performance.

Assess the unforced error and the mindset accompanying it.

Assessment should cover preparation, execution and impact at all levels. Self-reflection and self-assessment are crucial and help address the temptation to blame others.

Decide on a next best action for individual and team responsibility.

Map changes based on information, results, and feedback.

Author the corrective action, incorporating feedback and personal judgment.

Peter Drucker says that at this juncture, "Don't tell me what you're doing. Tell me what you stopped doing." An action plan may involve individual as well as team changes, because peak performance can be an individual and/or team endeavor. The transition from unforced error to successful accomplishment involves both undoing and doing, just as progress involves both unlearning and learning.

Program new identity.

Noel Tichy wrote in The Leadership Engine that a leader must have both the initiative and the courage to change the fundamental components of their business, if that will help the business evolve and remain viable. This fundamental aspect of identity incorporates individual as well as team performance. Each step of achievement needs to be metabolized as an evolving transformation of identity to become permanent.

Talent

A genius is not born but is educated and trained.
Laszlo Polgár

What is the role of talent in exceptional performance?

Laszlo Polgár rejected the notion of innate talent, emphasizing that deliberate practice and good habits could help a child become a genius in any field. He believed in hard, disciplined work and deliberate practice.

Polgár tested his theory with his three daughters Susan, Sofia, and Judit. He trained them in chess early on and raised them to become chess prodigies. Susan, the oldest, began playing chess when she was four years old, and was defeating adults within six months. Sofia, the middle daughter, was a world champion at fourteen, and became a grandmaster soon after. Judit, the youngest, was by age twelve the youngest player ever listed among the top hundred chess players in the world. Three years later, she became the youngest grandmaster of all time, besting previous record-holder Bobby Fischer. Judit was considered the strongest female chess player of all time.

To explore the talent myth, several in-depth studies were done on child prodigies, finding that those who seemed exceptional were in fact testaments to the 10,000-hour rule. They simply started earlier and trained harder. For example, in *Genius Explained*, Michael Howe found that Mozart had accumulated, with mentoring and intensive training by his father, at least 3,500 hours of practice by the time he was five years old. Similar stories featuring other gifted performers reveal the same intense exposure: Tiger Woods, the Williams Sisters and David Beckham.

A growth mindset realizes that talent can be enhanced through dedication and deliberate practice. A fixed mindset sees talent as either present or not, rather than as something that can be developed. Edwin Moses, winner of 107 consecutive foot races and four world records, said, “I ran against a lot of individuals who were probably more physically talented.”

We now know from several perspectives that talent is not a genetic gift but a developmental process. Fundamental talent, when present, can be enhanced when recognized, focused on and nurtured by parents, teachers, coaches and mentors. Discipline and deliberate practice evolve both intellectual and physical talents. The social setting and enhancing performance framework contribute to motivation as well.

To recognize and advance sports talent in leading pastimes is easy: baseball and basketball in the United States, soccer in England, ice hockey in Canada. Popular sports make it easy because they are so visible, identifiable, and measurable. Talent in other areas may not be as easily recognized. Talent in art, verbal ability, physical and mental skills can be challenging to identify and nurture.

The optimum model that evolved from various studies about the development of expertise and talent includes these aspects:

- Early diversification, sampling of a number of different activities.

- Exposure to informed choices, with long-term involvement.
- Later specialization, perhaps by mid to late adolescence.

Early diversification, the sampling of several activities, adds to the positive implications and exposure to result in both informed choices and long-term involvement. Deliberate play—for example, experiencing sport through enjoyable games—builds a foundation of intrinsic motivation. Deliberate play also establishes a range of cognitive and motor skills that help develop expertise and self-management.

Only later, experts suggest, perhaps by age thirteen, should specialization occur. It's not until late adolescence that children develop the physical, social, cognitive, emotional and motor skills needed to specialize in one sport or endeavor (Dr. Eddie O'Connor, *The Psychology of Performance*).

The notion that "all kids should be taught the skills for all positions" applies not only in sports, but in the intellectual and artistic pursuits needed for a basic developmental foundation. Achieving effectiveness and mastery in different areas builds a core identity that will persist for life. Many parents and some educators tend to push kids to do more of what they're already good at.

A composite of studies of elite performers across several fields identified a few common traits contributing to exceptional performance:

- The successful management of anxiety in pressure situations

- Confidence
- Mental toughness and resilience
- The ability to focus and block distractions
- A hard-work ethic
- The practice of setting and achieving goals
- Coachability
- Optimism

While there are certain genetic advantages in some areas of endeavor, we can influence the developmental process, which (depending on the endeavor in question) can have a far larger effect on performance. Discipline and deliberate practice are necessary, as well as the support and encouragement of others, family included.

Performance involves learning how to think and focus, understanding the context of the process, and focusing on the technical and tactical aspects of the endeavor. It's important to have "space" during this process. Crowding by parents, teachers, coaches or mentors can interfere with concentration and development.

Acknowledging progress and achievement is crucial. The key to any endeavor is to internalize the process until it becomes self-directed and self-sustaining, without input from others. Unconditional support from parents and others, including later colleagues and mentors, is an essential and valuable element. Children (and all learning individuals) are always taking unconscious notes about who they hope they can become, and how to get there from here.

Elite athletes and performers download the model of coaching and affirmation that later becomes their own template. Emotional regulation is best taught by modeling, and ultimately internalized for self-regulation.

A study of Olympic champions' parents found several common characteristics: keeping success in perspective, evaluating performance as opposed to outcome, teaching psychological skills, and focusing on values like hard work and commitment. Support and instruction included guidance on reacting to mistakes as well as handling remarkable success.

Parents and mentors are role models, perhaps the most important of all achievement influencers. Children (later proteges) watch and listen to how you respond. What you say (and don't say) matters. As parents, we don't know exactly what will be most important to our children, which means that everything is potentially important. The same is true of coaches and players. Framing mistakes as opportunities for growth supports the learning process.

The model of engaging in deliberate practice, developing and maintaining skills, and striving to achieve becomes a lifelong process, a template for engagement and achievement at each stage of transition. Aging athletes and intellectuals can still function and perform at their highest levels. What may be lost in one area can be made up for in another. Selective practice can aid in skill retention, and diminish age-related decline. Deliberate practice and goalsetting are constants throughout life. Commitment is reinforced by enjoyment and satisfaction.

Deliberate practice is difficult, relentless and repetitive work over a long period of time. Two of the "child prodigy" musicians I worked with took ten and fourteen years, respectively, to gain international recognition in their fields. Olympic gymnasts I've worked with took a similar period, with near-exclusive dedication to their skills. They and other top performers share some commonalities:

- Relentless dedication: commitment + grit
- A growth mindset
- Use of a series of coaches as their skills evolved
- Countless hours of repetitive practice
- Exclusive focus on specific performance skills
- Resilient focus despite boredom and lack of fun

The same framework (in a different context) underlies the success of executives and other professionals. Each is a creative and dedicated artist, whether business or professional. Each has learned that the surest path to consistent improvement involves constant practice, and a mindset focused on growth. These, in turn, build a commitment fueled by passion and framed by purpose.

Is there a disadvantage to talent?

The talent myth assumes a fixed mindset: why spend time and energy trying to improve, if success only comes to those with the right talents or genes? This is probably the most important reason to downplay the significance of innate talent (even though it can at times be a significant factor). The talent myth holds that innate talent is an all-important factor that determines outcome. The growth mindset recognizes that consistent effort can improve both skill and intelligence.

Talent can be a potential disadvantage, as someone with a natural talent may not at the very beginning of skill development subject himself or herself to the same hard work, rigors, and dedication as someone without those abilities. Natural talent can suffice for a period, but if it replaces the discipline and dedication to practice that needs to be developed, it can be a disadvantage. Those with less skill early on must work harder to develop it and may establish a systematic way to grow and improve in this process. They may also develop related skills to supplement their achievement, such as knowing their opponent, engagement strategies, and other adaptations. Without relying totally on natural athletic or intellectual capacity, they persevere through adversity to hone a foundation of repeatable strategies and skills.

A shadow story of talent is that it can mask poor teaching or coaching for a significant period and maybe even until it's time to play a bigger game in some challenging way, intellectually or physically.

Sustainable Success

It was insane. It was overwhelming. It was exciting. It was scary because that one thing that you don't get trained to do, like in drama school, they're not preparing you for success. They're preparing you to contend with failure. They're preparing you for resilience, and so when it all was said and done, I felt blessed that I made it without a nervous breakdown. Then it was like trying to figure out what my life was going to be after that.

Lupita Nyong'o, on winning an Oscar for Twelve Years a Slave immediately after graduating from the Yale School of Drama

Marcus Aurelius hired a servant to walk behind him as he made his way through the Roman town square, and the servant's only job was to whisper in his ear when people praised him, "You're only a man. You're only a man."

After their first whirlwind tour of the United States, The Beatles returned to England and immediately cut their next album. In fact, they did a new album every six months. They didn't take time off to bask in victory or allow success to derail their plans. Instead, they pressed their advantage and refused to let anything hijack their focus.

Dr. Mihaly Csikszentmihalyi, a pioneer in the field of positive psychology, also contributed to the study of creativity. Over the course of fifty years, he interviewed game-changing geniuses from diverse fields, including inventors, artists, Nobel Prizewinning scientists and Pulitzer Prizewinning writers. He discovered that creative geniuses spent their time intensely pursuing an activity, and then engaging in restoration and recovery. He found that this combination fosters breakthrough ideas and discoveries, while preventing creative burnout and cognitive fatigue.

Csikszentmihalyi discovered a common process among outstanding intellectuals and creative performers:

- Emerging: total engagement in their work.
- Incubation: a period of rest and recovery, when they didn't think about their work.
- Insight: new ideas and growth in their thinking.

Tough decisions and challenging mental tasks deplete energy and cognitive sharpness. Fatigue from one task spills over into another. For example, after someone exerts self-control, the prefrontal cortex activity diminishes, and this mental draining decreases self-control. The brain works much like the body. After lifting weights to the point of fatigue, arm muscles don't function very well. Likewise, after you've used your mind to the point of fatigue it, too, won't function quite so well. This fatigue may lead you to give up on solving tough intellectual problems, or to give in to other challenges.

The growth equation involves a balance of stress and rest. Deep talent must meet hard work with sustained passion. Maintaining success in any field is often as or more challenging than achieving that success in the first place.

Once you've achieved the pinnacle, how do you motivate yourself to continue the cycle of mental and physical endurance required to compete and excel the next time?

We now know that resilience, even to sustain the experience of peak performance, can be measured and taught. Creating success is a significant challenge, but sustaining success and staying at the top can be an even greater challenge.

Elite performers are not distracted by the victories or failures of others and instead focus on what they can determine. Elite performers become masters of mentalization. They are consistently self-directed and inner-focused, during practice and performance. Their ability to rebound from setbacks and defeats relies on an intense focus on specific goals and aspirations. At the same time, they sustain effort and energy through small, step-by-step achievements, and consistent focus on the next best thing and the next action.

We can learn a great deal from the systematic focus on the next step, the short-term goal. And, from learning to visualize the experience of effectiveness and mastery while at the same time having an internal map of major events and goals.

Elite performers celebrate their accomplishments without losing focus on what comes next. The mindset of optimism frames the focus on what can be achieved. The sense of "I can do something about this" pervades every situation. Any failure or setback becomes reframed as an opportunity to learn and improve. Every failure becomes information for the evolving development of the performance story narrative.

Extraordinarily successful people achieve because they pursue excellence through purpose, passion, and deliberate practice. Most of them struggle more than the average person, even after they've reached the top. Often, the satisfaction of success comes not from achieving goals, but from engaging and pursuing them in a satisfying way.

Those who achieve their dreams—whether athletes, performers, or businesspeople—can sustain happiness if they're able to focus on the next goal. This is not an addiction, but a growth mindset incorporating ideal achievement and contribution. A desire to evolve and contribute becomes a bedrock theme of all happy and sustained achievement.

A Final Note

Whatever is important to you, whatever it is you want to do—look at the system before the goal. Understand the patterns and principles that will help you reach your goals. Establishing a goal creates a map that tells you where you are and where you want to go and provides a way to measure your progress along the way. Focusing on the next step ensures steady progress toward mastery. Deconstructing a performance story into its basic elements allows you to know precisely what is working—and what to change, and how to implement that change (or even a new storyline).

If you justify putting off preparation for superb performance with the thought that you have plenty of time, think about Kobe. Lennon. Tupac. Whitney. Michael. Prince. Orbison. Kennedy. And far too many more.

Peak performance and winning are not about fame, money, or accolades. All of these are temporary. The pursuit of excellence is about purpose, and the experience of satisfaction, pride, and mastery.

Your performance is also your legacy. It is your contribution to the experience and memories of others—the download of the model that you offer for those who interact with you. Like your children, people are always taking unconscious notes while you are talking about or doing other things. It's the foundation of your identity passed on epigenetically to those who you touch, teach, and interface.

Epilogue.
Transactional and Transformational Coaches:
A Letter to My Favorite Coach

At the Special Olympics, a "hugger" is assigned to each special athlete to encourage, validate, and affirm for competing rather than for winning. As the starter fired the gun for nine athletes with mental or physical challenges in the hundred-yard dash, one boy tripped, fell, and began to cry. The eight other runners stopped and went back to where he was crying on the track. A boy with Down's syndrome sat next to him, hugged him, and said, "Are you feeling better now?" Then all nine athletes held hands and ran to the finish line as the entire crowd stood and applauded. This moment shows what is important in sports.

Transactional coaches focus on success strategies, goals, and winning. They emphasize the contribution of each team member's individual performance for team victory.

Transformational coaches: Transformational coaches focus on ideals, purpose, and growth to all someone can become. They help each team member develop game and life skills to become the best version of themselves. They change lives. And the team usually wins.

If you're really lucky, they come along once in a lifetime.

But that's enough.

My favorite coach of all time was James Pennington, a true transformational coach. He had a favorite phrase that became my "soul's code"—the spark that ignites a life calling: "Your mind is the most powerful thing in the world."

We won championships. And we learned, without even realizing it at the time, how to be better people.

No matter how upsetting the other team, the referee, or the bad call—I never heard Coach lose his composure or speak negatively to an official or another player. Today, that seems remarkable when I see coaches and players going off on referees, other players, and even teammates.

When one of us was upset about a referee's call, he simply said, "When the ref makes a bad call, he'll know it, so keep playing and he'll make it up to you."

He helped us focus on what we could determine and let go of what we couldn't.

I have not yet found an exception in any part of my life, parenting, or business to his repeated counsel: "Keep your eye on the ball, and your head in the game."

His most sobering, effective way to get my attention in a basketball game: "Davie, he's eating your sack lunch under those boards."

And even after finishing the 27th grade to practice medicine, his conditioning game plan is still the best prescription: "Run a cold. Run a fever."

When my daughter and son coordinated a surprise 50th birthday party for me, my daughter located Coach to make sure he was invited. They knew how important he is to me. Other special people were there: friends, family, colleagues, co-authors, professors. Coach was the best surprise. I remember every word of his comments to the attendees.

I dedicated to him a Training Curriculum and Client Workbook I created for licensed, Specialty-Certified Professional Coaches.

When I was growing up (as my daughter would say, "Dad, back in the day when you had wooden skis and wooden braces") it was unheard of for a guy to say to another guy, "I love you." My Dad, son, and Coach were the only guys who I later said those words to. Of course, it took me way too many years to say it to him even then.

The last story Coach and I shared was a letter to him. He gave me permission to pass it on here.

Hi Coach,

I hope you're doing great.

I think about you often and with tremendous fondness and respect for what I learned from you at a nodal time in my life.

I wanted to share with you some stories that I tell about you that will be published in training curriculum for performance coaches, and a book. I hope I have represented this in a way that you would approve and be proud of. I'm attaching some rough draft passages.

I regularly talk about you in various ways, passing on the lessons I learned from you about being a good human being, and fortunate enough to have you mentor and coach me.

Obviously, you're one of the two most important men in my development, and I have passed that on to the subsequent people in my life, beginning with my children, grandchildren, and stepdaughters. They know you through me. An entire new generation of professional mentor coaches know you through the curriculum dedicated to you.

Whenever I had any question about what to do, whether something was right, or how to proceed, the two people I had, one on each shoulder, were you and my favorite grandmother. I think you knew her: Nina Loudamy, who I called Mamie.

My two questions—if there was ever any doubt:

• "Could I tell this to Mamie?" If yes, it was a go.
• "What would Coach say?" Yes meant yes, no meant no.

I recall the couple of times you cared enough to drive me 20 miles to the nearest city with a doctor for treatment before a big game to be sure I was at my best. I loved those trips, to be able to visit with you personally. The same was true earlier with Mamie. I knew that if I ever got sick, she would be the person to come out to the farm to visit and bring a comic book. I think – but I am not absolutely sure – that this didn't lead to a sick day that could have been avoided.

At that time, I couldn't put into words the tremendous love and respect I had for you as a man and a coach. And words still aren't important enough.

You taught me winning and to see myself as a winner, as someone who could make a difference to be more.

You were a game-changer.

When you came to my 50th birthday surprise at my weekend ranch, that was one of the highlights of my adult life. In your reflections, rather than focusing on what you probably observed about how I didn't like to actually hit people in football, and how much I loved the basketball "No contact or it's a foul" you simply said, "Davie doesn't have a mean bone in his body."

However you cajoled or bribed to get me to be named to the All-State basketball team and game, I am deeply appreciative. I know that was you, not me.

I have come full circle in coaching my son and daughter's sports teams, practicing and teaching psychiatry and psychoanalysis for 25 years, to become a Professional Mentor Coach.

I have trained several thousand medical students, Psychiatry residents and Psychoanalysts, and 2,300 Professional Coaches, including life, wellness, and performance coaches. Each of them knows about you. Your legacy continues through them. And their clients.

You are remembered and live on each time those of us you touched recreate what you gave us.

Families, life, business, and sports are about stories. A hero is at the foundation of each.

You're mine.

I love you.

For comments, questions, and feedback: *dkrueger@mentorpath.com*

To schedule a brief discussion for Mentor Coaching: *www.MentorPath.com "Schedule Now"*

europe books

www.ingramcontent.com/pod-product-compliance
Ingram Content Group UK Ltd.
Pitfield, Milton Keynes, MK11 3LW, UK
UKHW041143300926
15471UKWH00012B/125

9 791256 971688